Dedication

I DEDICATE THIS BOOK to the worldwide Daniel Fast community who came together on *The Daniel Fast* blog and website. You have led me to deep and powerful truths about our Kingdom of God life as I researched answers to your questions and pondered your comments. You have encouraged me with your kind letters and messages of support. You have joined me with your virtual presence and financial support as we ministered to the men, women, and children in southern Africa. And you have taken my hand as we work together to let others know about the precious and powerful gifts available to the children of God through prayer and fasting.

I am honored to be a member of this community with you. Thank you, dear friends. While I can't list your individual names here, please know that I am truly grateful to you for making this book possible . . . I dedicate it to you. May the peace of Christ continue to overtake every part of your lives.

Contents

Before You Begin

THE DANIEL FAST includes a very healthy eating plan. However, please allow the Great Physician to work hand in hand with your earthly physician. Any time you enter into a significant change to your diet and exercise routines, it's a good idea to check with your health professional for his or her input.

Fasting should never harm the body. If you have special dietary needs—if you are pregnant or nursing, if you have a chronic illness such as cancer or diabetes, if you are a young person who is still growing or an athlete who expends more than typical amounts of energy on a regular basis—contact your health professional and modify the Daniel Fast eating plan in a way that is appropriate to meet your health needs.

Introduction

BE BLESSED, DEAR CHILD of the Most High God! You are about to enter into an exciting, life-changing spiritual adventure. Fasting is a powerful spiritual discipline designed by our Creator to draw us closer to Him, and the Daniel Fast is an experience for your whole person: body, soul, and spirit.

As I write these words, I am more convinced than ever that God has anointed the Daniel Fast to strengthen and empower His children for this period in the church's history. At a time when world systems are shaking, obesity and disease are at an all-time high, and the power of darkness seems stronger each day, I have seen miracles happen when people turn their hearts to God and consecrate themselves for a period of prayer and fasting.

The Bible instructs us to measure the quality of things by their fruit. Clearly, the Daniel Fast bears much good fruit as it changes lives toward goodness, faith, and health. I receive thousands of e-mails and messages a year from people whose lives have been forever altered during their Daniel Fast. And that's why I am so excited about the renewal of this biblical discipline that I believe is powered by the Holy Spirit and sanctioned by God.

Throughout Scripture, we find numerous men and women entering into times of fasting: Job, Jonah, Esther, Isaiah, David, Jeremiah, Daniel, Joel, John the Baptist, Jesus, Matthew, Mark,

Luke, John, and Paul. Fasting is interwoven throughout the Bible as a normal and acceptable practice in our faith. It's not a rule born out of church doctrine or tradition. Rather, as many men and women are discovering today, fasting is a tool created by the Father to help bring His children into closer communication and relationship with Him.

Keep in mind, fasting is about food. It's about restricting all or some foods for a spiritual purpose. While the origins of fasting are not definite, we do know that God ordered specific times when His people were not to eat certain foods. When God initiated the Passover—or the Feast of Unleavened Bread—as recounted in Exodus 12, He was very specific about the foods that should and should not be eaten. When Moses met with God on Mount Sinai (see Exodus 34), he ate no food and drank no water for forty days.

So just what is the Daniel Fast? In the first chapter of the book of Daniel, we learn of the young prophet's tensions over the differences between the Babylonian customs and his Jewish ways, and it had to do with food. Daniel refused to defile the body that he had set apart for the God of Abraham, Isaac, and Jacob. The food offered to him—meat and wine that had been dedicated to the Babylonian false gods—wouldn't do. So Daniel and his companions entered a partial fast (restricting food for a spiritual purpose) so they could remain true to their God.

Throughout the rest of the Bible, we find stories of men and women of God who fasted as part of their spiritual discipline. And today, preachers and Bible teachers still profess the need for fasting. But rare is the occasion when someone offers step-by-step instructions for how to do it.

I believe that's the ministry God has given me. After communicating with thousands of men, women, and teens about the Daniel Fast, I've discovered that what people want most is instructions. They don't just want to know *about* fasting, they also want to know *how to fast*. The purpose of this book is to guide you toward a successful Daniel Fast. I want you to learn how to fast so you can realize the great benefits this biblical discipline offers. In these pages you'll learn:

1. How fasting can help you draw closer to God

2. What questions to ask before embarking on an extended fast

3. How to establish a purpose for your fast

4. How to prepare for a Daniel Fast that will enrich your body, soul, and spirit

5. About the dietary restrictions in the Daniel Fast

6. How to prepare nutritious meals that comply with the Daniel Fast (including more than enough recipes for breakfast, lunch, dinner, and snacks on a twenty-one-day Daniel Fast)

7. What it means to walk in the Spirit as He is in the Spirit and how to make this choice for your own day-to-day life

8. How to begin to revamp your life and claim your citizenship in the Kingdom of God

9. How to complete a Daniel Fast and continue the new habits you've formed to make a positive difference in your life

10. How to incorporate prayer and fasting in your life as an effective tool for your spiritual growth

As you read these words, I hope you sense a stirring of great anticipation and excitement inside. You are about to embark on a spiritual encounter that will open doors of understanding, growth, and faith like you have never known. In the following chapters, I'm going to show you how to have a successful and effective fasting experience that will strengthen your personal relationship with Christ.

When you finish this book, you will be completely equipped for your Daniel Fast. And if you have a question that is not addressed or adequately answered here, I will show you how to find what you need. My mission is to do all I can to help you and other members of the body of Christ experience a successful Daniel Fast.

So get ready to learn about the Daniel Fast and see how it can serve you as you continue on your quest to seek the Kingdom of God, develop your faith, and grow in the love and knowledge of our amazing Father.

Be blessed in all you do.

Susan Gregory
The Daniel Fast Blogger
Susan@Daniel-Fast.com

Now may the God of peace Himself sanctify you completely;
and may your whole spirit, soul, and body be preserved
blameless at the coming of our Lord Jesus Christ.

— 1 THESSALONIANS 5:23

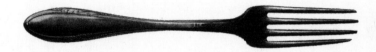

PART ONE

Sometimes you are so hungry, the only
way to be fed is to fast.

CHAPTER 1

Who Is the
Daniel Fast Blogger?

FIRST OF ALL, I'm not a preacher or a Bible teacher or a huge ministry leader. I am an ordinary woman whose life has been dramatically changed by stepping into a deeply personal day-to-day relationship with Jesus Christ. I've learned from my own experience and the experiences of others that we have a choice about how to live our lives. Jesus instructs us to seek the Kingdom of God and His righteousness (His way of doing things). God told His people that He has set before us life and death, blessings and curses, and He instructs us to choose life so that both we and our descendants may live. The choice is ours. And it's a choice with benefits that go beyond spending eternity with God. Thankfully, we can choose to have a dynamic, powerful, and purposeful life right here on earth and accomplish great things for God.

Every morning I make the choice to live a faith-driven life. I try to make every word I say and every action I take line up with the Word of God. Do I sound radical? Well, maybe I am, compared to a lot of people. I am radically alive with Christ, and the more

I focus my thoughts, activities, resources, and future on Him, the more exciting and at peace my life becomes.

I accepted Christ as a young woman and spent the next several decades participating in the typical activities of family, work, church, and social life. There were some great ups with family, motherhood, friendships, and achievements. And there were also some really tough downs, including an unwanted divorce and a long-term chronic illness. But I made it through those times with my mind and body still intact.

However, it wasn't until 2007 that I really started learning what living a life of faith is about. I was going through some really tough life experiences. It was the very beginning of the recession. My real estate investing business collapsed under the mortgage industry debacle and my finances were in shambles. I had no idea what I was going to do to even survive! Perhaps you've gone through that dark wilderness where hope seems so far away and relief seems out of sight. The pressure was on, and I felt utterly alone.

But I wasn't alone. I soon discovered the Bible's truth that Jesus will never leave us and will never forsake us. I learned that when we draw near to God He will draw near to us. I made a quality decision to believe everything in the Bible. I decided in advance that if doubt or fear reared their ugly heads, those would serve as signals that I needed to pursue more of the love and knowledge of Christ. Oh, He is so faithful! I set my mind on trusting God and His Word. I would get up every morning and spend hours studying faith and prayer. I wrote in my journal. I read books by well-respected and proven Bible teachers and preachers, spent hours talking with my Father, and proclaimed the truths and promises He made to His children.

It didn't happen overnight. It was like a big ship turning around—degree by degree, my doubt turned into faith and my fear turned into hope. I truly knew what it felt like to have the joy of the Lord as my strength. And through this process, my Father led me out of the wilderness and into His glorious light. The broken areas of my life began to heal, and as I purposed to build every part of my life on the Word of God, I entered into a life of stability, peace, and rest like I had never known before.

Part of this process was the Lord returning me to Christian writing. One day I was sitting on the couch in my living room. I wasn't meditating or praying or doing anything very "spiritual." I was just sitting. That's when I heard God's still, small voice in my spirit, *Start writing about the Daniel Fast.*

> "I began this fast fourteen days ago and all is well. I feel good spiritually, emotionally, and physically, plus I have lost ten pounds!
> —Corby "

That seemed like an interesting idea. I had practiced fasting for many years and was actually preparing to start a twenty-one-day Daniel Fast at the beginning of the New Year, which was just a couple of weeks away. I also had experience as a writer, although I had not written professionally for more than ten years. I searched the Internet and learned there wasn't a lot of information available about the Daniel Fast. Maybe there were others who needed to know more about this fast, and maybe I could help meet that need.

I knew from my own experience that many people begin the New Year with prayer and fasting. Since the start date was fast approaching, I had to get the information out quickly. I decided to write a blog titled *The Daniel Fast.*[1] Soon I had pages and pages of good information posted about the Daniel Fast, and it didn't take long until people started entering comments and asking questions on the blog. I replied to each one, and the comments and questions increased as the New Year approached.

After a few days, I quickly saw that the number one need of the people visiting the blog was recipes. So I scoured through my own recipe collection and began to adjust some to fit the Daniel Fast guidelines and make them available on my blog. This is when I could see God's plan unfold. Visitors to the blog were ecstatic to have the information they needed for a successful Daniel Fast, and I was launched into a whole new line of work. I could see that my loving Father had led me back into Christian writing for a sure purpose. Plus—and this is the big part—what I thought was merely a writing assignment, God meant for a lay ministry where I would meet the growing needs of His people.

Today, the blog has received more than 1.5 million hits, and I've been able to minister to thousands of men, women, and young people. I call myself the Daniel Fast blogger, but in reality, the title doesn't matter. I have experienced the grace of God in my life. My greatest ministry desire is to help men, women, and young people to learn to trust God and His Word more than anything.

Through this process, God has opened my heart to brothers and sisters in the body of Christ as they search for answers and practical instructions about this fasting practice. My great blessing is to serve God by serving His people. Many of the letters I receive from people bring me to tears as they share their victories during their Daniel Fasts. People who have never been successful at dieting have found victory as they focus on Christ and develop the fruit of the Spirit of self-control. I praise God with men and women who experience restored relationships with their spouses, parents, or children. Many write about answered prayer and miracles. And I especially love the testimonies about how people have learned for the first time to have an intimate and loving relationship with Christ.

Our God is so good, and He so wants His children to trust in Him and follow His ways so we can have the good life He planned for us. My number one goal is to help people experience a successful Daniel Fast so they can grow in the love and knowledge of our amazing Father and experience the love of Christ in new and remarkable ways.

The Bible teaches in James 4:8, "Draw near to God and He will draw near to you." Fasting puts us in a position to set aside a particular time when we can focus our attention on God and draw near to Him. In that nearness is the blessing and the power. In that nearness we experience God's presence and hear from Him. In that nearness we grow, work our faith muscles, and examine our hearts. The Daniel Fast offers you a Spirit-led opportunity to feed your soul, strengthen your spirit, and renew your body.

I am immeasurably thankful to the Lord for giving me this ministry, and with that blessing I truly want to be a blessing to others. I am honored that men and women are served with the information I share about the Daniel Fast. And I am thankful to you for entrusting me with the time and resources that you have invested in this book.

Please feel free to e-mail me at Susan@Daniel-Fast.com if you have questions that are not answered in these pages.

CHAPTER 2

Dusting Off an Ancient Spiritual Discipline

A GROWING MOVEMENT is taking place in the body of Christ. As individuals seek to feed their hunger for God, they've dusted off the ancient spiritual discipline of fasting. This is not a trend or a passing fad, but rather it is a rediscovery of a powerful way to access God in an intimate and authentic relationship, receive answers to prayers, and gain a fresh touch from our loving Father.

As we look to the Word of God, we see that almost every leader fasted. Prayer and fasting were typical in the Jewish spiritual life, and the people of the Bible knew the power of the practice. When they had great needs or were about to experience a great trial, they often sought God's wisdom and intervention through prayer and fasting. Consider the following:

- Moses: "So he was there with the LORD forty days and forty nights; he neither ate bread nor drank water. And He wrote on the tablets the words of the covenant, the Ten Commandments." (Exodus 34:28)

- Elijah: "So he arose, and ate and drank; and he went in the strength of that food forty days and forty nights as far as Horeb, the mountain of God." (1 Kings 19:8)

- Ezra: "Then Ezra rose up from before the house of God, and went into the chamber of Jehohanan the son of Eliashib; and when he came there, he ate no bread and drank no water, for he mourned because of the guilt of those from the captivity." (Ezra 10:6)

- Daniel: "I ate no pleasant food, no meat or wine came into my mouth, nor did I anoint myself at all, till three whole weeks were fulfilled." (Daniel 10:3)

- Esther: "Go, gather all the Jews who are present in Shushan, and fast for me; neither eat nor drink for three days, night or day. My maids and I will fast likewise. And so I will go to the king, which is against the law; and if I perish, I perish!" (Esther 4:16)

- Anna: "And this woman was a widow of about eighty-four years, who did not depart from the temple, but served God with fastings and prayers night and day." (Luke 2:37)

- Jesus: "Then Jesus, being filled with the Holy Spirit, returned from the Jordan and was led by the Spirit into the wilderness, being tempted for forty days by the devil. And in those days He ate nothing, and afterward, when they had ended, He was hungry." (Luke 4:1-2)

- Paul: "And he was three days without sight, and neither ate nor drank." (Acts 9:9) "In weariness and toil, in sleeplessness often, in hunger and thirst, in fastings often, in cold and nakedness." (2 Corinthians 11:27)

- Cornelius: "Four days ago I was fasting until this hour; and at the ninth hour I prayed in my house, and behold, a man stood before me in bright clothing." (Acts 10:30)

- Church leaders and elders: "As they ministered to the Lord and fasted, the Holy Spirit said, 'Now separate to Me Barnabas and Saul for the work to which I have called them.'" (Acts 13:2) "So when they had appointed elders in every church, and prayed with fasting, they commended them to the Lord in whom they had believed." (Acts 14:23)

As pressures of the present-day world increase, today's followers of Jesus Christ are seeking a deeper, more meaningful relationship with their Lord. They want a faith that goes beyond Sunday morning. They want their faith to make a difference in their families, their jobs, their everyday surroundings. They want to experience God in order to live a life that is Christ-centered, significant, and a positive witness to the world.

WHAT IS FASTING, AND HOW CAN IT BRING ME CLOSER TO GOD?

A growing number of Christians from every denomination have taken notice of the God-ordained discipline of fasting. Whether their fasts are corporate or personal, Christians are once again making this ancient practice a normal part of their spiritual routines.

Let's start with what fasting is and what it is not. First, fasting is always about food. The definition of a biblical fast is "to restrict food for a spiritual purpose." The Hebrew word for fast is *tsôwm* (tsoom) which means "to cover the mouth." The Greek word for fast is *nēstěuō* (nace-tyoo-o), which means "to abstain from food." Whenever fasts are mentioned in the Bible, they are accompanied with a spiritual issue. So when we consider biblical fasting, it always has to do with restricting food for a spiritual purpose.

Therefore, refraining from watching television or playing video games for a period of time might be a good decision, but it is not a fast. During a fast, many people choose to reduce the amount of time they give to certain pastimes or hobbies so they can devote more time to prayer, meditating on God's Word, or studying His ways. That's a great idea, as long as you realize that giving up specific activities is not a replacement for a true fast.

In addition to restricting or changing our eating habits, fasting always has to do with our spiritual life. Without that aspect, it's just a diet. Using the Daniel Fast eating plan for health purposes may be a good dietary change. However, understand that you would not be fasting if the spiritual component is not fully engaged. Imagine spending a day on the golf course. When you return to the clubhouse, someone asks how you did.

"Oh, I had a great day of golf," might be your reply.

When asked about your score, you reply, "Well, I didn't hit the ball today. I left my clubs in the car. But like I said, I had a great day of golf." The truth is that you may have had a very successful day walking and enjoying the grounds, but you were not golfing. The same is true with fasting. You may follow the eating plan with diligence and experience many great health benefits, but not including the spiritual component is like leaving your golf clubs in the car: you are dieting and not fasting.

This may come as a surprise to you, but fasting isn't for God. He's not going to think you are a better Christian or a more spiritual person because you fast. Your worth to God is totally dependent on Christ, who made you valuable and acceptable to the Most High God on the cross. So if you are fasting to prove to God how good you are, don't bother.

> My husband and I have absolutely loved the Daniel Fast. The meals are easy to prepare and very tasty.
>
> —D. R.

Instead, dear reader, fasting is for you. It's a spiritual tool that God created to help you strengthen your spirit, learn self-control of the flesh, draw closer to your Father, and focus on prayer. When you fast, you are stepping into a temporary set of actions for a spiritual purpose—like entering a bubble where everything is different for a set period of time. While you may gain some new disciplines while you fast and continue to practice them after you complete the fast, the experience is meant to be temporary because it is intense and with a specific purpose. There have been times when I have fasted and felt as if I was taking a crash course in spiritual matters.

When we study the Bible, we see that individuals are created in three parts. The Daniel Fast addresses each part of us. In 1 Thessalonians 5:23 we read, "Now may the God of peace Himself sanctify you completely; and may your whole spirit, soul, and body be preserved blameless at the coming of our Lord Jesus Christ." In Hebrews 4:12 we learn, "For the word of God is living and powerful, and sharper than any two-edged sword, piercing even to the division of soul and spirit, and of joints and marrow, and is a discerner of the thoughts and intents of the heart."

Some theologians say that we are spirits, we have souls, and we live in our bodies. We will look at this idea as it relates to the Daniel Fast in chapter 4.

Three types of fasting

Three types of fasts are mentioned in the Bible:

- An *absolute fast* is what Moses did when he was on Mount Sinai for forty days. The Bible recounts the fast in Exodus 34:28, "So he was there with the LORD forty days and forty nights; he neither ate bread nor drank water. And He wrote on the tablets the words of the covenant, the Ten Commandments." Rarely is an absolute fast practiced for a long period of time. Some will abstain from all food and all water for a short period of fasting, perhaps during daylight hours. But longer periods are not recommended since physical complications with long-term consequences could result.

- A *normal fast* is when only water is consumed. This would be the type practiced by Elijah (see 1 Kings 19:8) and Jesus (see Matthew 4). While we can't be absolutely sure that Elijah and Jesus abstained only from food for forty days, the accounts indicate that Elijah went without food but makes no mention of water and Christ was hungry with no mention of thirst.

- A *partial fast* is when some foods are consumed but others are restricted, which was the case of Daniel and John the Baptist. Most of us recall the story of John the Baptist, who survived only on locusts and wild honey (Matthew 3:4).
(I can see why the John the Baptist Fast hasn't captured the attention of today's Christians. There isn't a big demand for locusts!)

It seems that Daniel fasted frequently, with three of his experiences recorded in the book of Daniel. One was a normal fast as recorded in Daniel 9:3, when the prophet set his "face toward the Lord God to make a request by prayer and supplications, with fasting, sackcloth, and ashes." However, there are two other accounts when Daniel engaged in a partial fast, abstaining from some food, but not all.

In Daniel 1:12 we read that Daniel and his companions ate only vegetables, or pulse (KJV), which referred to foods that came from seeds, and drank only water. Then in Daniel 10:3 the prophet tells us, "I ate no pleasant food, no meat or wine came into my mouth, nor did I anoint myself at all, till three whole weeks were fulfilled." These are both partial fasts. The Daniel Fast is a partial fast modeled after the fasting experiences of the prophet.

Called fasts and corporate fasting

A *called fast* is a set time of fasting. For example, Lent is a called fast and the tradition of many Christian churches throughout the world. Lent has a start date and an end date. Many followers of Christ choose the Daniel Fast as their method of fasting during Lent.

Likewise, Passover (or the Feast of Unleavened Bread) is a called fast commemorating the Hebrews' escape from enslavement in Egypt. It is a partial fast and always begins on the fifteenth day of the month of Nisan, which is the first month of the Hebrew calendar. Passover was designed and established by God in Exodus 12 and is still acknowledged by Jews to this day.

A growing tradition among Christians today is to start the New Year with prayer and fasting, and many churches throughout the world call their members together for a period of *corporate fasting* at this time. From what I hear from visitors to *The Daniel Fast* blog and website, the most common is a twenty-one-day period, starting on the first Sunday after New Year's Day. And from the tens of thousands of site visitors every January, it's clear that many people participating in this corporate New Year fast use the Daniel Fast as their method of fasting because it's a partial fast and appropriate for their lifestyles.

> My husband enjoyed the fresh foods and whole grains that I served while fasting. We are looking forward to continuing to eat foods that are healthy for our family. —*Amy*

Similarly, throughout the year, churches and causes encourage their members to join in corporate fasts for a specific period of time. Again, when the fasting period is longer than three or four days, it appears that many people use the Daniel Fast as their method of fasting.

Fasting with a purpose

Since the definition of fasting is to restrict food for a spiritual purpose, before you start your fast, you'll want to be specific about your aim.

If you are joining your church community or a ministry in a corporate fast, then the leadership decides the purpose. For example, for years Jentezen Franklin, who is the pastor of churches in Gainesville, Georgia, and in Irvine, California, has championed a fasting movement every January to honor and seek God for the New Year. Lou Engle is the founder of TheCall, a ministry that organizes Christians for corporate prayer and fasting for issues concerning the United States. Several times each year they call for periods of prayer and fasting for specific issues such as racism, sexual immorality, and abortion. If you join a corporate fast, you will want to pray for the specific issues your leaders address, as well as matters in your own personal life.

A common purpose for fasting is to draw closer to God. This is an intentional choice to "turn down the noise of the world" and focus on your relationship with your Father. You may want to target one or two areas, such as prayer or hearing God's voice. You can then gather study materials prepared by reputable men and women of God who have learned and practiced these ways in our faith.

I entered my first fast in the early 1990s after a colleague told me of his positive fasting experience. He gave me a book by Arthur Wallis titled *God's Chosen Fast*. I read the paperback and began to fast for three days, drinking only water. I continued to fast periodically whenever I had special needs in my life. But in 2005, fasting took on a much deeper meaning for me. That was the first time I began the New Year with a twenty-one-day Daniel Fast.

Since that time, as I've experienced the value and yield of fasting, I've begun to practice this discipline several times a year. And I always start the New Year with a twenty-one-day Daniel Fast. Long before the fast commences, I begin to seek God's direction for my life and to hear His instruction for me for the upcoming months. Last year I was awakened in the middle of the night on January 1 by the Lord saying, *This is your year of transformation.* I felt as if a charged wave of hope entered my body! He was calling me to focus my attention for a full year on radical change under His direction.

As I entered the period of prayer and fasting, I kept that message at the forefront of my mind. During that time, the Lord showed me that I had merely settled for too many things in my life and that I needed to get extreme about attacking them! These weren't changes that could take place in just a few weeks. God wanted to take me to a higher level, and this was my *year* of transformation. The changes concerned my health, my home, my finances, and my ministry. He even showed me that I needed to focus only on these four areas so that I could give them all the required attention, study, time, and resources necessary to make a major change.

As you determine the purpose for your fast, I suggest you follow these steps:

1. Ask the Holy Spirit to show you your purpose. He is faithful when we ask for His help. I have often found that He fulfills my requests within one or two days.

2. Identify the top three or four issues in your life that cause you stress or concern. Ask yourself, *If I could change three things about my life, what would they be?*

3. Then present these needs to God for His intervention and direction during your fast.

WHAT IS THE DANIEL FAST?

The Daniel Fast is a partial fast in which some foods are restricted. It's a biblically based fast fashioned on the experiences of the prophet Daniel. Remarkably, the Daniel Fast has become one of the most popular forms of fasting, perhaps because it is not as demanding or daunting as eating nothing for many consecutive days. Instead, the eating plan for the Daniel Fast is similar to a vegan diet (completely plant-based with no animal products), though somewhat more restrictive.

The Daniel Fast is based on Jewish fasting principles and the experiences of the prophet in Daniel 1 and Daniel 10. In Daniel 1:12 we read Daniel's request to the steward, "Prove thy servants, I beseech thee, ten days; and let them give us pulse to eat, and water to drink" (KJV). Pulse was food that originated from seed, including legumes and fruit. Daniel also requested that they drink only water. This reference is what anchors the Daniel Fast as a plant-based eating plan with the only beverage being water. Since the diet is totally plant based, no animal products are consumed including fish, shellfish, dairy products, or eggs.

In Daniel 10:3 we learn that during a time of great mourning, Daniel also abstained from meat, "pleasant" food, and wine. It's on the basis of this account that we eliminate sweeteners, candy, and desserts from the Daniel Fast, along with alcohol—even in recipes. Sweeteners excluded during the Daniel Fast include sugar, honey, agave nectar, Stevia, cane juice, and syrups.

Because Daniel was a man of God, we can assume that he also followed Jewish fasting principles. In preparation for Passover, Jewish people removed all leavening products from their homes and did not include them in recipes. So during the Daniel Fast, all leavening products are eliminated, including yeast, baking powder, and baking soda.

Lastly, all the food on the Daniel Fast is natural, which eliminates man-made chemicals, artificial flavorings and colorings, food additives and preservatives, and highly processed foods. We also use no stimulants, including caffeine.

Detailed lists of foods to include and to avoid on the Daniel Fast can be found beginning on page 99.

LENGTH OF THE DANIEL FAST

There is not a definite period of time when you should engage in the Daniel Fast, nor is there a predefined number of days. Many people use this method of partial fasting for as few as seven days; however, to gain the health benefits of the fast, I've found that a longer period is better. It seems that most people use the Daniel Fast for a twenty-one-day period, partly because that's what the prophet did in Daniel 10:2 and also because many corporate fasts are called for a twenty-one-day period. I have used the Daniel Fast for as few as ten days and for as many as fifty.

The length of your fast can be determined by the leaders of a corporate fast or by promptings from the Holy Spirit. One time I was fasting for a three-week period. I completed the fast, but the very next day I was prompted to continue fasting for two more weeks. So I advise you to follow the leading of the Holy Spirit if you are not sure about how long to fast.

ARE YOU READY?

Even though you can eat during the Daniel Fast, it is no less effective than a complete fast. The power in fasting has less to do with food than with setting yourself apart for a specific period of time to focus more on the Lord, prayer, and worship. In other words, the power of fasting is found when you consecrate yourself to the Lord and discipline yourself to focus on Him. That's how your spiritual experience is enhanced.

Don't get me wrong. There is sacrifice and discipline involved in the Daniel Fast. Though eating meals consisting of fruits, vegetables, whole grains, nuts, and seeds may not seem difficult, you *will* have your battles! The cravings begin when you give up all sweeteners, caffeine (probably the hardest for most people), all beverages except water, leavened breads, chemicals, and deep-fried foods. But that's all part of the fasting experience as you overcome the flesh by denying it the food it craves.

> The past three weeks have been an amazing journey. I truly appreciate the recipes and words of encouragement.
> —*Angela*

Your period of prayer and fasting should be different from your typical days. Think about how you approach a vacation. It's also a distinct time in your life. You prepare for your vacation to make sure everything is in order. And while you are vacationing, you have very specific goals, whether they be relaxation, new experiences, or a separated time with your family and friends. You do different activities on your vacation as you experience this set-apart time.

Similarly, your fast is a distinct time that will be different from your usual days, so you will want to prepare for it. Just like you enter into a period of vacation, you will enter into your fast. You will do different activities, and you will have specific goals.

Over the last few years, I have found that the benefits of fasting can be known only through the experience itself. I like to tell people that the Daniel Fast is for the whole person: body, soul, and spirit.

- Your body will benefit from the healthy eating plan.
- Your soul (your emotions, intellect, and feelings) will benefit from the spiritual discipline of fasting.
- Your spirit will grow in strength and in the knowledge of Christ and His ways.

The power of fasting doesn't necessarily make sense to the natural mind. But spiritual fasting requires spiritual sense—a spiritual outlook and trust in the Lord and His ways. Starting a Daniel Fast is the first step toward an experience that will bring you closer to the Father who desires a deep, abiding relationship with each of His children. Are you ready to cross that threshold? Are you prepared to join with thousands of others who are longing for a deeper, more effective life with God? Are you looking for an encounter with the Almighty?

If you are, then it's time to learn about the Daniel Fast.

CHAPTER 3

Daniel—Determined to Live for God in Enemy Territory

OUR MODEL for the Daniel Fast is a renowned man of God who lived more than 2,700 years ago. Even though he is considered an ancient prophet, his life is an excellent example for us to consider as we face the challenges in our world today. Take the time in the next day or two to read through the book of Daniel. It won't take long to peruse the twelve chapters, and as you do, you will quickly notice the stark contrast between those who put their trust in the God of Abraham, Isaac, and Jacob and those who chose worldly gods and idols. You also may detect the parallels that exist between the Babylonian system of Daniel's day and the world you and I live in right now.

Daniel was raised in Jerusalem and was likely from an upper-class or royal Jewish family. He would have been steeped in the traditions and customs of the Hebrew people, including their religious practices. Throughout the Scriptures we find references to the "customs of the Law." These were the common religious practices that all those of faith followed, including Daniel.

The Hebrew people meticulously followed these customs, which in turn shaped their lives and developed their faith and commitment to God. It's important to know that these valuable customs didn't stop when Jesus delivered our new covenant. In fact, Christ and His family followed the customs of the law as well. When Jesus was just eight days old, His parents took Him to the Temple for a customary ritual in which baby boys are circumcised and parents announce the name they have selected for their child.

And when eight days were completed for the circumcision of the Child, His name was called Jesus, the name given by the angel before He was conceived in the womb. —LUKE 2:21

Have you ever wondered what is so important about the eighth day? I see our loving God all over this custom. The baby is presented and named in the house of the Lord on the eighth day because the mother is considered "unclean" for seven days after the birth of her child. By waiting until the eighth day, she is able to be present for this important ceremony.

> " I am happily on my fourth day and I am finding myself full, even with hardly anything to eat.
>
> —*Nicole* "

You can see how the customs and laws were deeply ingrained in the daily lives of the Jewish people in biblical times. This included the daily prayers, which are cited many times in the book of Daniel. These prayers helped to keep him close to God even though he was in captivity.

Three prayer services were recited daily: *Shacharit*, from the Hebrew *shachar*, which means "morning light"; *Mincha* or *Minha*, the afternoon prayers named for the flour offering that accompanied sacrifices at the Temple in Jerusalem; and *Arbith* also called *Arvit* or *Ma'ariv*, meaning "nightfall."

According to the Talmud, which is the book of rabbinical law, prayer is a Biblical commandment drawn from Deuteronomy 11:13, "to love the LORD your God and serve Him with all your heart and with all your soul." The phrase "with all your heart" is a reference to prayer. According to the Talmud, there are two reasons for having three basic prayers. First, to recall the three daily sacrifices at the Temple in Jerusalem. And second, because each of the patriarchs instituted one prayer: Abraham the morning, Isaac the afternoon, and Jacob the evening. These prayers were read aloud and followed by the faithful:

- **Daniel** followed the custom: "Now when Daniel knew that the writing was signed, he went home. And in his upper room, with his windows open toward Jerusalem, he knelt down on his knees three times that day, and prayed and gave thanks before his God, as was his custom since early days." (Daniel 6:10)

- **King David** followed the custom: "Evening and morning and at noon I will pray, and cry aloud, and He shall hear my voice." (Psalm 55:17)

- **Anna** followed the custom: "Now there was one, Anna, a prophetess, the daughter of Phanuel, of the tribe of Asher. She was of a great age, and had lived with a husband seven years from her virginity; and this woman was a widow of about eighty-four years, who did not depart from the temple, but served God with fastings and prayers night and day." (Luke 2:36-37)

- And **God** referred to the custom when He instructed Joshua: "This Book of the Law shall not depart from your mouth, but you shall meditate in it day and night, that you may observe to do according to all that is written in it. For then you will make your way prosperous, and then you will have good success." (Joshua 1:8)

Daily prayer was not an option for God's chosen people; it was a commandment. Children were raised with these Jewish customs, so following them was simply part of their lives. Daily prayer and reading from the Scriptures kept the Word of God in their minds and in their hearts. Again, we see Jesus following the customs that had been passed down through the generations:

> *So He came to Nazareth, where He had been brought up.* And as His custom was, *He went into the synagogue on the Sabbath day, and stood up to read.* —LUKE 4:16, EMPHASIS ADDED

In the late sixth century BC, Nebuchadnezzar was conquering so many kingdoms that he needed more able men to fulfill his edicts throughout his empire. That's when he raided Jerusalem for their best and most qualified people.

> *Then the king instructed Ashpenaz, the master of his eunuchs, to bring some of the children of Israel and some of the king's descendants and some of the nobles,* young men in whom there was no blemish, but good-looking, gifted in all wisdom, possessing knowledge and quick to understand, who had ability to serve in the king's palace, *and whom they might teach the language and literature of the Chaldeans.*
> —DANIEL 1:3-4, EMPHASIS ADDED

What Nebuchadnezzar didn't know was that although he was taking the noble young men away from Jerusalem, he could not take away the truth of God's Word that had taken root in their hearts.

There are two valuable lessons in this example. One is the wisdom in God's instruction to parents as recorded in Proverbs 22:6: "Train up a child in the way he should go, and when he is old he will not depart from it." And the second is the immeasurable value of daily prayer. Three times each day, Daniel planted seeds into his heart from the Word of God. God's commandments were at the forefront of his mind. He did not depend on his own way of thinking, nor was he swayed by the practices of his captors. Instead, God's truth gave him direction and confidence.

My prayer for you as you engage in this period of prayer and fasting with the Daniel Fast is that daily prayer will become your custom, just as it was for David, Daniel, Joshua, Anna, and others who had a deep and abiding faith in their God. They serve as our models for living a God-centered life, and we can choose to follow their examples.

Daniel's commitment to God was unwavering. He knew who he was, and he wasn't about to let his captors corrupt him. When Daniel and his companions were first brought to Nebuchadnezzar's palace, the king gave strict instructions that these prized slaves were to eat the very best food. He had big plans for them, and he wanted them to be strong, fit, and well cared for. These noble young men were to eat the same food that was served to the king!

But Daniel refused the food for a couple of reasons. First, the king's meat and wine had been offered to the Babylonian gods; and second, the Jewish people had strict laws about how meat was to be prepared. To eat or drink the king's foods would require Daniel to step over a line he wasn't willing to cross.

But Daniel purposed in his heart that he would not defile himself with the portion of the king's delicacies, nor with the wine which he drank; therefore he requested of the chief of the eunuchs that he might not defile himself. —DANIEL 1:8

Daniel "purposed in his heart" to follow the ways of God. This wasn't a spur-of-the-moment decision. Instead, it was an offshoot of the course Daniel had established for himself from the time he was very young. He was a man of God, and therefore he would behave according to the ways of his Lord.

What was it Daniel wanted to avoid? He didn't want to defile his body. That means that he had already submitted his body and soul to his God. He was under the law, and he didn't want to do anything that would not be consistent with the ways of the Lord.

So Daniel bought some time as he negotiated a plan with the

chief of the eunuchs: "Please test your servants for ten days, and let them give us vegetables [pulse or food grown from seed] to eat and water to drink. Then let our appearance be examined before you, and the appearance of the young men who eat the portion of the king's delicacies; and as you see fit, so deal with your servants" (Daniel 1:12-13, definition added).

This request is one of the components of the Daniel Fast. We see here that Daniel ate only foods grown from seeds and drank only water. Some translations say he ate only "vegetables" and drank only water. According to Matthew Henry, the highly respected Bible scholar, pulse was a common reference to foods that come from seeds rather than from animals.[2] So the reference to vegetables most likely was translated from "pulse" and included fruits and other foods that come from seeds of the ground.

> It's day six and I'm hanging in there. I'm actually enjoying the discipline of being reminded how much my physical wants drive my behavior. —Jackie

As the account continues, we learn the outcome. Daniel and his companions ended up having superior health compared to the others that did not follow God's ways. Plus, when Nebuchadnezzar spent time with the young men, he found them to have more wisdom and understanding than all those in his realm: "As for these four young men, God gave them knowledge and skill in all literature and wisdom; and Daniel had understanding in all visions and dreams" (Daniel 1:17). The Hebrew men were superior, not because of a position or rank that was awarded to them, but because of who they were—men shaped by the ways of the Lord.

Throughout the book of Daniel, you will find accounts of how these four men faced struggles and challenges without fear. Why? They were confident in their God and His powers. They led disciplined lives and fed their hearts with the Word of God day and night.

Daniel and the others grew in stature and power. They were regularly acknowledged for their integrity, wisdom, and skills, and their promotions stirred the jealousy of the others serving the king.

When Daniel was promoted to preside over the leaders the king set in place, some searched out ways to sabotage him.

They were especially incensed when they learned that the king was considering putting Daniel over the whole empire, like a prime minister: "Then this Daniel distinguished himself above the governors and satraps, because an excellent spirit was in him; and the king gave thought to setting him over the whole realm" (Daniel 6:3).

Though the governors and satraps had set their minds on knocking Daniel off the pedestal, they couldn't find any grounds to bring charges against him. That's when they devised a plan to coerce the king into signing an irretractable thirty-day edict to forbid prayer to anyone but the king: "All the governors of the kingdom, the administrators and satraps, the counselors and advisors, have consulted together to establish a royal statute and to make a firm decree, that whoever petitions any god or man for thirty days, except you, O king, shall be cast into the den of lions" (Daniel 6:7).

Remember Daniel's custom of daily prayer? Remember his resolve to live his life for God and follow His commandments? He wasn't about to change under this or any other pressure:

Now when Daniel knew that the writing was signed, he went home. And in his upper room, with his windows open toward Jerusalem, he knelt down on his knees three times that day, and prayed and gave thanks before his God, as was his custom since early days. —DANIEL 6:10

Daniel followed the custom of daily prayers that were recited aloud. And as you can see in this passage, Daniel's prayers could be heard through the open window. Praying the Scriptures aloud was part of the custom of the Jewish people in the Old Testament times and also in the New Testament:

Now an angel of the Lord spoke to Philip, saying, "Arise and go toward the south along the road which goes down from Jerusalem

*to Gaza." This is desert. So he arose and went. And behold, a
man of Ethiopia, a eunuch of great authority under Candace
the queen of the Ethiopians, who had charge of all her treasury,
and had come to Jerusalem to worship, was returning. And sitting in his chariot, he was reading Isaiah the prophet.*

—ACTS 8:26-28

The story goes on to explain that Philip heard the man reading
Isaiah. He was practicing the custom of the law to read the Scriptures aloud. The Ethiopian eunuch wasn't reading to himself, he
was proclaiming the Word of the Lord. If you have never done this,
I encourage you to read the Scriptures aloud on a daily basis, just as
the Jews of old did. You will soon find faith stirring in your spirit
as the powerful Word of God is spoken into the surroundings and
sinks into your heart.

For Daniel, reading aloud had some consequences: he was
arrested. And even though the king valued Daniel very much, he
couldn't go against his own law. So Daniel was doomed to the den
of lions. But again, Daniel had the Word of God deeply rooted in
his soul. He had faith in God that His promises were true.

The king was sickened by this crisis. After Daniel was thrown
into the lions' den, the king went back to his palace and was so
worried that he couldn't sleep. Early the next morning, he rushed
to the lions' den to see if Daniel had survived. Daniel's response
serves as a powerful example for you and me.

*Then Daniel said to the king, "O king, live forever! My God sent
His angel and shut the lions' mouths, so that they have not hurt
me, because I was found innocent before Him; and also, O king,
I have done no wrong before you." Now the king was exceed-
ingly glad for him, and commanded that they should take Daniel
up out of the den. So Daniel was taken up out of the den, and
no injury whatever was found on him, because he believed in his
God.* —DANIEL 6:21-23

Do you see that last phrase?—"because [Daniel] believed in his God." That's the kind of faith we can have! A faith so strong that nothing can harm us! But the question is, are we willing to do what Daniel did in order to have what Daniel had? Are we willing to love God with our whole hearts? Are we willing to read the Scriptures and pray three times each day? Are we willing to truly make God number one in our lives? So many times we can't figure out why our prayers are not answered or why there is so much stress and unrest in our lives. Daniel never wrestled with these issues because he was always filled up with the truth of God.

> " I finished eating my Vegetarian Chili. I felt like I was doing something wrong because it was just too delicious!
> —*Sheila* "

I think it's important to note that God didn't keep Daniel from ever entering the lions' den, just like he didn't keep Daniel's companions from being thrown into the fiery furnace (see Daniel 3). But God met them in the midst of their calamities and delivered them. And in this account, we see that the reason Daniel was delivered is "because he believed in his God."

Dear reader, this serves as a challenge and invitation for each of us. Daniel didn't start cramming his heart with Scriptures when he found out he was going to be thrown in the lions' den. And he didn't sit inside the cave crying and begging God to save him. No, Daniel had the faith he needed *before* his enemies ever started conspiring against him. He had his armor on—and he kept it on all the time.

Finally, my brethren, be strong in the Lord and in the power of His might. Put on the whole armor of God, that you may be able to stand against the wiles of the devil. For we do not wrestle against flesh and blood, but against principalities, against powers, against the rulers of the darkness of this age, against spiritual hosts of wickedness in the heavenly places. Therefore take up the whole armor of God, that you may be able to withstand in the evil day, and having done all, to stand. —EPHESIANS 6:10-13

God is more than willing to do His part when we are willing to do ours. He has given us everything we need to live a fulfilled and purposeful life. Our Lord never speaks of failure for us; He is our victory. Jesus says, "These things I have spoken to you, that in Me you may have peace. In the world you will have tribulation; but be of good cheer, I have overcome the world" (John 16:33).

But a victorious life comes by faith, and our faith is activated by the Word of God. It's a spiritual principle that cannot be broken. It is not a legalistic guarantee that we will live a victorious life because we stuck with a read-through-the-Bible-in-a-year schedule. We will have that victorious life when the Word of God penetrates our hearts and God is able to reveal His truths to us.

Daniel grew old in Babylon, and he had many more amazing experiences as his faith in God was confronted and the power of God worked through him. His life was not unusually protected and honored because God gave him special privileges. Instead, he lived his love unto the Lord, and therefore he received all the favor and privileges available from our God.

You and I have a lot in common with Daniel and the other Hebrew men. As believers, we are also in enemy territory, facing the pressures of this world. And just like Daniel, we can chose to live our lives according to God's ways—not just when it's convenient and not in a casual way. If we want what Daniel had, we must be willing to do what Daniel did. He devoted himself to God. He set his heart on the ways of the Lord and refused to be defiled by the customs and practices of the Babylonians.

Daniel's faith brought him through. His life lived for God is why you and I are even giving him attention today! And his life of unwavering faith is why he serves as a worthy example for us as we enter into a powerful period of prayer and fasting unto the Lord.

CHAPTER 4

The Daniel Fast for Body, Soul, and Spirit

BECAUSE THE DANIEL FAST confronts each of our three parts[3]— body, soul, and spirit—this discipline helps us to understand in a greater way how God created us. Several years ago, I discovered some powerful details about our human makeup that led to a profound change in my life and opened my understanding of the Word of God and the principles of the Kingdom. It was like the lights turned on for me and I could see more clearly. And the more I've come to understand the three-in-one makeup of our beings, the easier it has been for me to live a life of faith unto the Lord.

It all started when I attended the Sunday morning adult Bible study at my church. We were working through the book of Hebrews. Ron Stokes, our facilitator, is a retired army officer who has several graduate degrees and is a "seasonal accountant," meaning that during tax season he works for a local firm to prepare people's filings. As you might imagine, Ron was very detailed and organized. He is passionate about the Word of God and was particularly gifted in leading our class in a verse-by-verse study of Hebrews. I especially enjoyed those times when we "hung out" on one verse and gleaned powerful truths from God's living Word. That's what happened when we reached Hebrews 4:12:

> *For the word of God is living and powerful, and sharper than any two-edged sword, piercing even to the division of soul and spirit, and of joints and marrow, and is a discerner of the thoughts and intents of the heart.*

Though the verse was familiar to me, I had never spent time tearing it apart and looking into its deeper meaning. This was my opportunity. A few days later, in my quest for understanding, I got out my trusty yellow pad and printed my name at the top. Then I drew three simple stick figures to represent the three parts of me.

You may have heard the description, "You are a spirit, you have a soul, and you live in a body." The Word of God mentions our three-in-one makeup in 1 Thessalonians 5:23:

> *Now may the God of peace Himself sanctify you completely; and may your whole spirit, soul, and body be preserved blameless at the coming of our Lord Jesus Christ.*

In the Bible, the soul is often referred to as "the flesh," and I realized that even though I had been a Christian for decades, too often my flesh was in authority over my spirit rather than the other way around! The Bible calls it living with the "carnal mind." Consider the following:

- Paul wrote in 1 Corinthians 3:1-3, "And I, brethren, could not speak to you as to spiritual people but as to carnal, as to babes in Christ. I fed you with milk and not with solid food; for until now you were not able to receive it, and even now you are still not able; for you are still carnal. For where there are envy, strife, and divisions among you, are you not carnal and behaving like mere men?"

- Romans 8:6 says, "For to be carnally minded is death, but to be spiritually minded is life and peace."

- In 2 Corinthians 10:4 we learn, "For the weapons of our warfare are not carnal but mighty in God for pulling down strongholds."

- And in Colossians 3:1 we are told, "If then you were raised with Christ, seek those things which are above, where Christ is, sitting at the right hand of God."

This was one of those times when God revealed His truth directly to me. In the Greek, the word for "dividing or separating" as used in Hebrews 4:12 is *merismos*. I could understand the separation of my spirit and flesh—my *merismos*—as never before by looking at the little stick figures. So I made a decision to walk in the Spirit rather than be ruled by my own flesh. I would submit to the Lord and the Holy Spirit would be in control.

This teaching also led me into a much better understanding of what "walking in the Spirit" is all about. There are attitudes of the Spirit and attitudes of the flesh. When I feel pride, resentment, or other "fleshly" emotions arise in me, I quickly can see that it is my flesh "acting out." I can then get a grip and choose to walk in the Spirit.

Other attitudes of the Spirit and flesh include the following:

Spirit	Flesh
love	pride
forgiveness	resentment, bitterness, hate
faith	fear
selflessness	ego, self-centeredness
humility	arrogance, jealousy
self-control	lust

This is just a partial list, but I think you can get the idea. Christ calls us to walk according to the Spirit and not the flesh. We are to crucify our flesh—all those worldly thoughts and emotions—and allow the Holy Spirit to guide us and direct us.

That's the way Daniel and his companions lived their lives. They were sold out to God and they filled their minds, hearts, and words with Him and His ways. When Nebuchadnezzar threatened to throw Shadrach, Meshach, and Abed-Nego into the fiery furnace, their faith was so strong they didn't even flinch:

> *Shadrach, Meshach, and Abed-Nego answered and said to the king, "O Nebuchadnezzar, we have no need to answer you in this matter. If that is the case, our God whom we serve is able to deliver us from the burning fiery furnace, and He will deliver us from your hand, O king. But if not, let it be known to you, O king, that we do not serve your gods, nor will we worship the gold image which you have set up."*   —DANIEL 3:16-18

This wasn't a faith built from Sunday morning church attendance and prayers over their meals. This was a deeply rooted faith in God they had developed by filling their souls with God's Word and truth on a daily basis.

If you want a Spirit-led life, if you want to explore more about yourself and the way that God made you, the Daniel Fast can help you do that. But first, let's go a little deeper! Let's gain even greater understanding and start "in the beginning." Try to picture these scenes in your mind:

> *Then God said, "Let Us make man in Our image, according to Our likeness; let them have dominion over the fish of the sea, over the birds of the air, and over the cattle, over all the earth and over every creeping thing that creeps on the earth." So God created man in His own image; in the image of God He created him; male and female He created them. Then God blessed them, and*

God said to them, "Be fruitful and multiply; fill the earth and subdue it; have dominion over the fish of the sea, over the birds of the air, and over every living thing that moves on the earth."
—GENESIS 1:26-28

When God created Adam and Eve, they were completely integrated beings. They walked and talked with God, and His Spirit was alive and well in them. Life was good! Even God agreed:

Then God saw everything that He had made, and indeed it was very good. —GENESIS 1:31

We all remember God's instruction to man: "Then the LORD God took the man and put him in the Garden of Eden to tend and keep it. And the LORD God commanded the man, saying, 'Of every tree of the garden you may freely eat; but of the tree of the knowledge of good and evil you shall not eat, for in the day that you eat of it you shall surely die'"(Genesis 2:15-17).

Adam and Eve were closely connected to God. The Word says that He walked with them in the cool of the day. They had everything they needed for life—and it was good! Really good!

However, we also remember the result of Adam and Eve not heeding God's instruction. They were deceived by the slithering enemy of God and ate the fruit. Consequently, they died. But they didn't die physically, because Adam went on to live until he was 930 years old and Eve was the mother of several children. While they didn't die physically, they did die spiritually. No longer were they in sync with God. Instead, through their disobedience, the nature of the enemy was now in their soul. And their sin was passed down through their offspring and through the ages, even to you and me. Romans 5:12 says, "Therefore, just as through one man sin entered the world, and death through sin, and thus death spread to all men, because all sinned."

As a result of their choice to disobey God, the tree of life, the fruit of which Adam and Eve could freely eat—was no longer available to them. Their access to the Garden was blocked, and they could no longer partake of heaven and all God had for them. God had given Adam authority over the earth, and through his disobedience, Adam relinquished this control to Satan, who is now known as "the god of this world" (2 Corinthians 4:4, KJV). Adam was cut off from the perfect life he had with God.

> *So He drove out the man; and He placed cherubim at the east of the garden of Eden, and a flaming sword which turned every way, to guard the way to the tree of life.* —GENESIS 3:24

Picture the three parts of our makeup aga in. Adam's spirit had been alive, but because of his sin it died. The part that still existed in Adam—his soul with its intellect, feelings, and emotions— was now separated from God. Faith died and worldly reason took its place. We might call this reason "common sense" or "living a moral life." But without God's wisdom, that life is still doomed. Proverbs 14:12 puts it this way: "There is a way that seems right to a man, but its end is the way of death."

That separation from God and the sin we inherited from Adam are still present when human beings enter this world. Each life is born with a living body and soul, but with a dead spirit. Psalm 51:5 says, "Behold, I was brought forth in iniquity, and in sin my mother conceived me." So when you and I came to this earth, instead of being born with a live spirit, we were born with a soul that was separated from God, a sinful nature.

> "Without your advice on prayer and Scripture, this would have seemed like a boring diet. Adding the Lord makes all the difference in the world.
>
> —*Barbara*

The Creator was grieved by this separation, and for centuries He wooed His people toward Him. Over and over again He sent prophets and angels to teach His people to follow His ways so they could have a good life.

Now let's fast-forward to Bethlehem, more than four thousand years after Adam and Eve were evicted from the Garden of Eden. Picture this in your mind: an angel of the Lord appeared before the shepherds keeping watch over their flocks. He told them they would find a baby wrapped in swaddling clothes, lying in a manger. Then suddenly, just as this birth announcement left the angel's lips, his words were joined by an outburst of worship by a multitude of the heavenly host praising God, saying, "Glory to God in the highest, and on earth peace, goodwill toward men!" (Luke 2:14).

The Savior, God's reconciliation to humanity, had arrived! Now there was finally a way for our spirits to come to life.

> *For God so loved the world that He gave His only begotten Son, that whoever believes in Him should not perish but have everlasting life. For God did not send His Son into the world to condemn the world, but that the world through Him might be saved.*
> —JOHN 3:16-17

Because of Jesus, we can be redeemed and reunited with God our Creator, and the Kingdom of God is open to us again! Of course this news would bring out the heavenly hosts.

So how does this all happen? Jesus explained the process to Nicodemus:

> *There was a man of the Pharisees named Nicodemus, a ruler of the Jews. This man came to Jesus by night and said to Him, "Rabbi, we know that You are a teacher come from God; for no one can do these signs that You do unless God is with him."*
>
> *Jesus answered and said to him, "Most assuredly, I say to you, unless one is born again, he cannot see the kingdom of God."*
>
> *Nicodemus said to Him, "How can a man be born when he is old? Can he enter a second time into his mother's womb and be born?"*
>
> *Jesus answered, "Most assuredly, I say to you, unless one is*

born of water and the Spirit, he cannot enter the kingdom of
God. That which is born of the flesh is flesh, and that which is
born of the Spirit is spirit. Do not marvel that I said to you,
'You must be born again.' The wind blows where it wishes, and
you hear the sound of it, but cannot tell where it comes from and
where it goes. So is everyone who is born of the Spirit."

—JOHN 3:1-8

As you study the Word of God, you will see that the only way for our spirits to be redeemed and regain open access to God is through Christ.

Jesus said to him, "I am the way, the truth, and the life. No one
comes to the Father except through Me." —JOHN 14:6

You may have heard the line, "Many paths lead to God." It may be politically correct, but it's just not the truth. Jesus says *no one comes to the Father except through Him.* The reconciliation of our relationship required a blood sacrifice. Jesus became that sacrifice for us, paying the price so that we could be reconciled with God. Our Holy God cannot be in the vicinity of unholy beings. He cannot be with or even near sin. So to restore us, we must be blameless. The blood of Jesus makes that possible.

Our spirits must be reborn so we can come into full relationship with God—and the only way for that to happen is through Jesus. Even Jesus had to wrestle with this fact. When He was in the garden of Gethsemane, "He went a little farther, and fell on the ground, and prayed that if it were possible, the hour might pass from Him. And He said, 'Abba, Father, all things are possible for You. Take this cup away from Me; nevertheless, not what I will, but what You will'" (Mark 14:35-36).

But Jesus knew the priceless value of His shed blood. The only way our spirits could be born again and we could be reconciled to our Father was through Jesus' sacrificial and agonizing death:

*And being in agony, He prayed more earnestly. Then His sweat
became like great drops of blood falling down to the ground.*

—Luke 22:44

So when we accept the free gift of Christ—when we choose to
unite ourselves with God by making Christ our Savior—we are
born *again*. Why *again*? Because though our spirits were already
created at the beginning of the world, they died because of sin.
Now our spirits can be born again because of the saving and sacrificial blood of Jesus Christ. We come alive in Christ and are grafted
into Him as John 15:5-8 tells us:

*I am the vine, you are the branches. He who abides in Me, and
I in him, bears much fruit; for without Me you can do nothing. . . . . By this My Father is glorified, that you bear much
fruit; so you will be My disciples.*

We are His branches and as we submit ourselves to Him, He is
able to work through us so that we can bear much good fruit. And
the good fruit we bear glorifies our Father.

I get so excited about this! Are you ready for more? Here we go!

Picture the scene when John the Baptist baptized Jesus. As soon
as Jesus came up out of the water, the Holy Spirit descended and
immediately drove Jesus into His first spiritual battle. Our Lord
was quick to start taking dominion back from the enemy. He prepared Himself in the wilderness with forty days of fasting. And
then He confronted the wicked one. Seeing he wasn't making any
ground, Satan left (waiting for a better opportunity), and the angels
came and ministered to Jesus.

Shortly thereafter, Jesus returned to Galilee to tell people about
a whole new life that was available to them.

*The time is fulfilled, and the kingdom of God is at hand. Repent,
and believe in the gospel.* —Mark 1:15

For most of my Christian life I missed the amazing truth of this proclamation. I didn't realize what Jesus was talking about. Jesus was not just saying, "Be remorseful for your sins, people. Say you are sorry so you can go to heaven." Though that's clearly part of what we must do, it's far from the whole Good News. Sadly, most people don't understand the complete picture.

Instead of announcing a ticket to heaven, Jesus was announcing a new way of life—an everlasting life that starts here and now. He was saying, "Repent!" which means "change." He was, and still is, telling everyone who will listen to Him that a new day has dawned. For thousands of years, direct access to God had been blocked. But Jesus made the way open to us. He reconciled us to our Father. He also opened the doors back to the Kingdom and the tree of life. And the Kingdom of God reality is different from the world we have known. "For through Him we both have access by one Spirit to the Father. Now, therefore, you are no longer strangers and foreigners, but fellow citizens with the saints and members of the household of God" (Ephesians 2:18-19). The chains of sin have been broken. An amazing new world is available to us—a new way of thinking, believing, and behaving. A new way of living is at hand. It's the Kingdom of God, and we are invited to be a part of it.

> " I was on the Daniel Fast just for a week. But that week was amazing! The closeness with God was so awesome that I can't describe it.
>
> —Sheila "

Remember when the disciples asked Jesus to teach them to pray? Jesus instructed them to say, "Your kingdom come. Your will be done on earth as it is in heaven" (Matthew 6:10). The walls are broken! All has been restored, and because of Jesus we again have access to the tree of life Adam had lost. Hebrews 4:16 tells us, "Let us therefore come boldly to the throne of grace, that we may obtain mercy and find grace to help in time of need."

Do you see this? When Jesus was praying to God before His crucifixion He said, "I have given them your word. And the world hates them because they do not belong to the world, just as I do not belong to the world. I'm not asking you to take them out of the world, but to keep them safe from the evil one. They do not belong to this world any more than I do" (John 17:14-16, NLT).

As followers of Jesus Christ and children of the Most High God, we are citizens in the Kingdom of God. It's a place that operates on a different set of principles and spiritual laws, all of which are activated by faith.

Jesus answered, "My Kingdom is not an earthly kingdom. If it were, my followers would fight to keep me from being handed over to the Jewish leaders. But my Kingdom is not of this world."
—JOHN 18:36, NLT

When we come into life with Christ, everything changes for us! Prior to our rebirth, we were brought up under the world's system and understanding. But with Christ all things are new, and it is through Him and the Word of God that we learn the ways of this Kingdom. Jesus said, "I am the *way*, the *truth*, and the *life*. No one comes to the Father except through Me" (John 14:6, emphasis added).

Jesus is the only access to the truth about God:

Don't let anyone capture you with empty philosophies and high-sounding nonsense that come from human thinking and from the spiritual powers of this world, rather than from Christ. For in Christ lives all the fullness of God in a human body. So you also are complete through your union with Christ, who is the head over every ruler and authority. —COLOSSIANS 2:8-10, NLT

I hope you can grasp the amazing truth of what God has done for us. He loves each and every one of us so much that He gave what was most valuable to Him—His Son. And why? So we could be in seamless fellowship with Him once again, so that His original plan for all of humanity could be restored, and so we could be saved from an eternity of being separated from God—which is hell!

Every single person ever born in this world will exist forever. When we exhale our last earthly breath, we will pass on to another realm, another kingdom. That's where we will live forever. *Forever*—it's a very long time—it's endless time. But because of Jesus, you and I have the choice as to which kingdom we will spend eternity in. With Jesus you can live in the Kingdom of God, where love rules and everything is perfect—nothing missing, nothing broken! Only good will surround you. Or you can live in the kingdom of darkness, where all of God's goodness, mercy, and nature are absent.

The good news is that you are still breathing today, and you can make a decision right now to choose your future address. If you have never asked Jesus into your heart, you can do it right now as you're reading these pages! It's as simple as a four-sentence prayer: "Jesus, I am sorry for turning my back on You all these years. Today, I want to choose the everlasting life my Creator wants me to have. Please forgive me of all my past wrongs. I invite You into my heart and ask You to be my Lord and my Savior."

That's it! If you were sincere with that simple prayer, your spirit just came to life and you are a new creature in Christ. All is brand-new, and Jesus just took up residence in your heart. You may not feel any different, but believe me, you are very much changed! If you like, e-mail me at Susan@Daniel-Fast.com and tell me you accepted Christ. I'll send you some information about how to begin this amazing faith-driven life.

Wow! I feel like doing the Happy Dance. Now let's take a closer look at each individual part of our makeup, the things that make us who we are: the soul, the spirit, and the body.

THE SOUL

The soul is referred to by many other names in the Bible, including the flesh, the natural man, and the old man. The Bible teaches, "For he who sows to his flesh will of the flesh reap corruption, but he who sows to the Spirit will of the Spirit reap everlasting life" (Galatians 6:8).

The soul is the nonmaterial part of you that was born from the egg of your mother and the "seed," or sperm, of your father. It's the seat of your conscience, emotions, personality, intellect, and will. Does the soul have value? Oh, yes! God loves every soul that was ever created. He sent His Son to save our souls and redeem us into what God had planned us to be in the very beginning. But the unredeemed soul can never enter the Kingdom of God and have everlasting life.

Before the birth of Christ, people "behaved" their way into a right standing with God. History shows that they weren't very good at it on their own. In fact, before the great Flood, humankind was so corrupt and far from God that He saw no hope in their future (see Romans 1:18-32).

And the LORD was sorry that He had made man on the earth, and He was grieved in His heart. —GENESIS 6:6

God started over with Noah and his offspring to repopulate the world and fulfill the vision our Creator had for us. He put this family in a large boat along with animals of every kind and destroyed the people who had reached such reprehensible levels.

So even though a new age with new inhabitants was started, they still did not have the Spirit of God living in them. So how did they know what was right and what was wrong? Through the law that later came from God to Moses and from Moses to God's chosen people. The apostle Paul teaches a lot about the law, but it can seem very complex. *The Message* makes Paul's point somewhat easier to understand:

But I can hear you say, "If the law code was as bad as all that, it's no better than sin itself." That's certainly not true. The law code had a perfectly legitimate function. Without its clear guidelines for right and wrong, moral behavior would be mostly guesswork.

Apart from the succinct, surgical command, "You shall not covet,"
I could have dressed covetousness up to look like a virtue and
ruined my life with it.

Don't you remember how it was? I do, perfectly well. The
law code started out as an excellent piece of work. What hap-
pened, though, was that sin found a way to pervert the com-
mand into a temptation, making a piece of "forbidden fruit"
out of it. The law code, instead of being used to guide me, was
used to seduce me. Without all the paraphernalia of the law
code, sin looked pretty dull and lifeless, and I went along with-
out paying much attention to it. But once sin got its hands
on the law code and decked itself out in all that finery, I was
fooled, and fell for it. The very command that was supposed to
guide me into life was cleverly used to trip me up, throwing me
headlong. So sin was plenty alive, and I was stone dead. But the
law code itself is God's good and common sense, each command
sane and holy counsel.

I can already hear your next question: "Does that mean
I can't even trust what is good [that is, the law]? Is good just
as dangerous as evil?" No again! Sin simply did what sin is so
famous for doing: using the good as a cover to tempt me to do
what would finally destroy me. By hiding within God's good
commandment, sin did far more mischief than it could ever
have accomplished on its own. —ROMANS 7:7-13, THE MESSAGE

Praise God that we have been redeemed by faith in the blood of
the Lamb. We don't have to find our way to God's grace by following the law. Romans 3:28 says, "Therefore we conclude that a man
is justified by faith apart from the deeds of the law."

The soul cannot perceive truths from the Spirit of God:

But the natural man does not receive the things of the Spirit
of God, for they are foolishness to him; nor can he know them,
because they are spiritually discerned. —1 CORINTHIANS 2:14

The apostle Paul puts it this way in his letter to the Christians in Corinth, "If the Good News we preach is hidden behind a veil, it is hidden only from people who are perishing. Satan, who is the god of this world, has blinded the minds of those who don't believe. They are unable to see the glorious light of the Good News. They don't understand this message about the glory of Christ, who is the exact likeness of God" (2 Corinthians 4:3-4, NLT).

Until the spirit is alive, a natural man (not yet born again) cannot understand or make any sense of the things of God. They are foolishness to him. However, as born-again Christians with Christ alive in us, we can submit our whole beings to God, as we learn in Romans 12:1-2:

> *I beseech you therefore, brethren, by the mercies of God, that you present your bodies a living sacrifice, holy, acceptable to God, which is your reasonable service. And do not be conformed to this world, but be transformed by the renewing of your mind, that you may prove what is that good and acceptable and perfect will of God.*

Your soul can be transformed to the degree that you renew your mind, change your attitudes, and conform to the Word of God. This transformation of the mind is maturing in Christ, and it's an ongoing process. But it doesn't happen automatically—even when the spirit is reborn. The renewing of your mind is the result of a voluntary act of submission.

Daniel lived every day in submission to the Holy God. He didn't have a "microwave" faith, but rather a faith steeped in consistent prayer and worship:

> *Now when Daniel knew that the writing was signed, he went home. And in his upper room, with his windows open toward Jerusalem,* he knelt down on his knees three times that day, and prayed and gave thanks before his God, as was his custom since early days. —DANIEL 6:10, EMPHASIS ADDED

Daniel's way of life—his lifestyle—was centered on God. He had a reputation as a man filled with the Spirit. He had conquered pride and developed his faith so it could be seen by everyone in Babylon and used by his God.

THE SPIRIT

The spirit is our innermost part. It is the God-centered essence where Christ abides. Remember, the spirit is different than our body (or flesh). Jesus addressed these two parts in John 3:6 (NIV), "Flesh gives birth to flesh, but the Spirit gives birth to spirit." Your mother didn't provide the egg for and give birth to your spirit. And your father didn't provide the seed of your spirit. Only God can give birth to your spirit. As the Bible tells us:

> *Having been born again, not of corruptible seed but incorruptible, through the word of God which lives and abides forever.*
>
> —1 PETER 1:23

When we receive the "seed" of Christ through the Word of God, our spirits are born of the Spirit. That's why we are called children of God! And all God's children are made righteous by the blood of Christ. Nothing else would work in God's presence.

The curse from Adam's sin is broken when we accept Christ:

> *Therefore, as through one man's offense judgment came to all men, resulting in condemnation, even so through one Man's righteous act the free gift came to all men, resulting in justification of life. For as by one man's disobedience many were made sinners, so also by one Man's obedience many will be made righteous.*
>
> —ROMANS 5:18-19

Once again, as a child of the Most High God, you are a spirit, you have a soul, and you live in a body. All three parts of you are active and experiencing life on earth. But which part is in control? Our physical body doesn't have a mind of its own. So we need to look at our spirit or our soul to see which part of us is running things.

We've all been in a spot where we know we *should* do one thing, but we don't follow that wisdom and we make a different choice. Even the disciples had to learn this. Look at Jesus' words of warning to His disciples in the garden of Gethsemane:

> *Then He came to the disciples and found them sleeping, and said to Peter, "What! Could you not watch with Me one hour? Watch and pray, lest you enter into temptation. The spirit indeed is willing, but the flesh is weak."* —MATTHEW 26:40-41

The apostle Paul also wrestled with this issue: "I don't really understand myself, for I want to do what is right, but I don't do it. Instead, I do what I hate" (Romans 7:15, NLT). Why is this part of the human condition? Again, the Bible explains it all: "For the flesh lusts against the Spirit, and the Spirit against the flesh; and these are contrary to one another, so that you do not do the things that you wish" (Galatians 5:17).

The soul is where our feelings camp out. Feelings are good at following, but not at leading. Can you imagine letting your feelings lead your life? "Oh, I don't feel like going to work today." Or "I feel so good in new clothes! I'm going on a shopping spree even though I don't have the money for it." Or "That person hurt my feelings! I'll never talk to him again!"

In order to learn to walk in the Spirit, we need to put Him in the leadership role and then let our feelings provide the joy, laughter, and sense of calm that accompanies a life lived according to God's plan. Here is how we do just that:

> *My old self has been crucified with Christ. It is no longer I who live, but Christ lives in me. So I live in this earthly body by trusting in the Son of God, who loved me and gave himself for me.*
> —GALATIANS 2:20, NLT

Walk in the Spirit, and you shall not fulfill the lust of the flesh.
— GALATIANS 5:16

The benefits of living a Spirit-led life are immense, "There is therefore now no condemnation to those who are in Christ Jesus, who do not walk according to the flesh, but according to the Spirit" (Romans 8:1).

Another amazing thing about all this is that when we walk according to the Spirit, we have access to all God's power and spiritual resources!

Let us therefore come boldly to the throne of grace, that we may obtain mercy and find grace to help in time of need.
— HEBREWS 4:16

We can't access the throne of God when we're in the flesh. But when we are walking in the Spirit, then all of heaven is open to us. Listen to what Jesus told His disciples about the coming of the Holy Spirit into their lives:

But now I go away to Him who sent Me, and none of you asks Me, "Where are You going?" But because I have said these things to you, sorrow has filled your heart. Nevertheless I tell you the truth. It is to your advantage that I go away; for if I do not go away, the Helper will not come to you; but if I depart, I will send Him to you. And when He has come, He will convict the world of sin, and of righteousness, and of judgment: of sin, because they do not believe in Me; of righteousness, because I go to My Father and you see Me no more; of judgment, because the ruler of this world is judged.

I still have many things to say to you, but you cannot bear them now. However, when He, the Spirit of truth, has come, He will guide you into all truth; for He will not speak on His own authority, but whatever He hears He will speak; and He will tell you things to come. He will glorify Me, for He will take of what is Mine and declare it to you. All things that the Father has are Mine. Therefore I said that He will take of Mine and declare it to you. —JOHN 16:5-15, EMPHASIS ADDED

Now that our spirits have been born again, we have a divine connection with the Holy Spirit! Isn't that amazing? I hope some of these familiar verses are lighting up for you in a new way as you begin to really grasp who you are in Christ.

Living with Christ is living in the Spirit, and we live in the Spirit through faith:

> *For I am not ashamed of the gospel of Christ, for it is the power of God to salvation for everyone who believes, for the Jew first and also for the Greek. For in it [the good news of Christ—the gospel] the righteousness of God is revealed from faith to faith; as it is written, "The just shall live by faith."* —ROMANS 1:16-17

So we need to make a choice as to whether the Holy Spirit will have control over our beings or we will give those reins to the flesh. Way back in Deuteronomy, when God was showing the Israelites the life they could have if they obeyed Him rather than following their own ways, God's people were given a choice as to how they could live their lives:

> *See, I have set before you today life and good, death and evil, in that I command you today to love the LORD your God, to walk in His ways, and to keep His commandments, His statutes, and His judgments, that you may live and multiply; and the LORD your God will bless you in the land which you go to possess. But if your heart turns away so that you do not hear, and are drawn away, and worship other gods and serve them, I announce to you today that you shall surely perish; you shall not prolong your days in the land which you cross over the Jordan to go in and possess. I call heaven and earth as witnesses today against you,*

that I have set before you life and death, blessing and cursing; therefore choose life, that both you and your descendants
may live; *that you may love the LORD your God, that you may
obey His voice, and that you may cling to Him, for He is your
life and the length of your days; and that you may dwell in the
land which the LORD swore to your fathers, to Abraham, Isaac,
and Jacob, to give them.*

—DEUTERONOMY 30:15-20, EMPHASIS ADDED

We have a choice about how we are going to live our day-to-day
lives. We can walk in the Spirit or in the flesh. We can choose to forgive . . . or we can hold grudges. We can gossip about people . . . or
we can choose to speak only good words about others. We can snap
at a store clerk . . . or we can give grace and mercy. We can trust in
God with our lives and walk in faith . . . or we can depend on ourselves and the world systems.

I truly believe that a lot of Christians suffer from unanswered
prayer because they are still walking in the flesh, rather than walking in the Spirit. Though they are saved and their spirits are alive,
they have not made the conscious choice to walk in the Spirit
where they have access to God and His power. God connects with
our spirit, not with our flesh.

Again, think back to Daniel. He was a devoted man of God,
even when facing extreme pressure and torment. Nothing could
sway him because he trusted God. And God never failed him—
God was faithful to Daniel, and God is faithful to you and me.

During the Daniel Fast, you will be confronted over and over
again with the choice whether to give the power over to the Holy
Spirit or to let your flesh have its way. You will be faced with countless choices. Sometimes the choice will be about your body. Will
you exercise today or stay in bed an extra thirty minutes? Is your
spirit in control or your flesh? Sometimes it will be about your attitude. Will you walk in the Spirit while you're at work or with your
family members? Sometimes it will be about how you will use your

time. Will you plan your day so God can be first? Or will you surf the Internet for hours or watch television sitcoms?

These choices provide valuable discipline in building up your faith, and this is where fasting can serve as a training ground for your whole being. During your fast, you will have to put the Holy Spirit in charge, forcing your flesh and your body to submit to the ways of the Spirit. The Holy Spirit will help you make choices about what to eat and how much. The Holy Spirit will guide you to get up in the morning and what you will do. And during this time of consecration (separating yourself for a spiritual purpose) the Holy Spirit will help you to be diligent about opening yourself to God so He can teach you and minister to you. Then your spiritual ears will be sharpened so you can hear God speak to your heart.

I hope you are feeling excited! Your fast truly can be a life-changing experience as you learn more about living a Kingdom of God lifestyle and as you open yourself to the supernatural power of His resources. As you fast, concentrate on developing your faith and letting the Holy Spirit teach and guide you into all the things that are yours as a child of God.

> "I am trying to wean myself from Diet Coke this week. I have not had one! That is a huge feat in itself.
> —*Norma*"

THE BODY

The body is easy to understand. You can see it! It is the physical place where our spirit and soul reside. Some people call it our "earth suit." But the physical body is also an amazing part of our being. God told Jeremiah, "Before I formed you in the womb I knew you; before you were born I sanctified you; I ordained you a prophet to the nations" (Jeremiah 1:5).

David praised the Lord with these words:

For You formed my inward parts; You covered me in my mother's womb. I will praise You, for I am fearfully and wonderfully

made; marvelous are Your works, and that my soul knows very
well. —PSALM 139:13-14

During the Daniel Fast, your body will come under the control of your spirit. At first, it might try to rebel as you change the
foods you've been feeding it. Perhaps the greatest uprising comes
to those who have been feeding their body caffeine every morning! I can hear my rebellious body now, "What, you're not going to
give me the pick-me-up I've become accustomed to each morning?
Well, I'll show you. Here's a dose of fatigue, and I'll even throw in
a couple of headaches and a few leg cramps to let you know I'm not
too thrilled about this change! I liked your coffee habit!"

The good news is that your body will soon thank you for the
changes and pay you with powerful dividends of energy, clear
thinking, and vitality. Those are good rewards!

I'm not a health professional, but I am a great admirer of these
amazing physical dwellings that God created for us to inhabit. Like
all of His creation, I am stunned by the beauty, inventiveness, wonder, and functionality of our human bodies!

I also love reading new scientific discoveries that prove what the
Bible has been telling us all along! For example, Dr. Caroline Leaf,
a learning specialist who has spent more than twenty-five years
studying the brain and the way we think, writes:

Thoughts are real things: they have a structure in your brain
and occupy space. Thoughts are the same as memories.
Thoughts and memories look like trees and are called neurons
or nerve cells. You build a double memory of everything as a
mirror image of each other. This means that the memory on
the left side of the brain builds from the detail to the big picture; and the memory on the right side builds from the big
picture to the detail. When you put these two perspectives
of thought together, you get intelligent understanding taking place. As information comes in from the five senses, you

process it in certain structures of your brain, then you grow branches on the "trees" to hold this information in long term memory. In fact, as you are reading this, you are growing thoughts, because, thoughts are the result of what we hear and read and see and feel and experience. This means that whatever you grow is part of you, actual branches in your brain that create your attitude and influence your decisions.[4]

In her book *Who Switched Off My Brain?* Dr. Leaf explains why good health is critical to do what the Bible says in 2 Corinthians 10:5: "bringing every thought into captivity to the obedience of Christ." When negative thoughts are allowed to stay in our thinking, they literally grow into toxic elements that can bring us harm. Dr. Leaf also explains that there is actually a thinking mechanism in our physical hearts. As the rapid-speed thought process works, forces are going into our heart and back to our brain as part of the decision-making process.

Our bodies are truly wonderful and declare the glory of God, which is just one of the reasons we should take good care of them. In 1 Corinthians 6:19, this question is asked of us: "Or do you not know that your body is the temple of the Holy Spirit who is in you, whom you have from God, and you are not your own?"

Our bodies are valuable vessels because God resides in us! And He wants to accomplish great and important things through us. He wants us to be healthy, able, and ready warriors so we can carry out the purpose for which we are called. Jesus says, "You did not choose Me, but I chose you and appointed you that you should go and bear fruit, and that your fruit should remain, that whatever you ask the Father in My name He may give you" (John 15:16). You were born for this very time, and God has a special and important appointment for you. You are needed and highly valuable!

We need to be in good condition—our spirits, our souls, and our bodies! We are members of a great and powerful family. And all members are needed, worthy of their assignments, and unique to fulfill the call God has on their life.

We are not our own. So when we abuse our bodies with unhealthy living, we are not at our best. We are not being good to ourselves, those around us, or our Lord. He needs us to be strong and healthy warriors who bring glory to Him.

The Daniel Fast serves as an excellent tool to help you bring your body into alignment with your Creator's intention for you. You can feed it good quality foods in healthy portions and in balanced meals. You can make sure your body is well hydrated by drinking plenty of filtered water each day and forgoing sweet and chemical-laden beverages that do it harm. You can make sure your body gets adequate exercise by walking and stretching. You can make sure your body is rested by giving it adequate sleep and relaxation. And perhaps one of the most important things you can do for your body is to do your very best to live a stress-free life by depending on God and walking in His ways.

The Daniel Fast provides a way to feed our souls, strengthen our spirits, and renew our bodies. It is modeled after one of our greatest prophets. And many witnesses are quick to testify about the amazing changes that have happened while they have set themselves apart for a focused time of prayer and fasting.

This is your opportunity. Welcome to the Daniel Fast. May this powerful discipline bring you into a mighty relationship with your Father.

CHAPTER 5

Five Steps for a Successful Daniel Fast

I HAVE BEEN BLESSED through the Daniel Fast ministry to communicate with thousands of people throughout the world. For many, I guide them into their first fasting experience. For others, I share in their upcoming or current fast. Through this, I have been able to identify five specific steps each person can take toward a rewarding fast.

1. **Pray.** From the very beginning, include God in your fast. Open yourself up to Him and talk to Him about your intentions. Submit the fast and yourself to Him. If you are not accustomed to this type of interaction and intimacy with the Lord, that's okay. He understands. But keep moving forward, even though you might feel awkward. Remember, He knows what you need before you tell Him. The psalmist writes, "O LORD, You have searched me and known me. You know my sitting down and my rising up; You understand my thought afar off. You comprehend my

path and my lying down, and are acquainted with all my ways. For there is not a word on my tongue, but behold, O Lord, You know it altogether. You have hedged me behind and before, and laid Your hand upon me. Such knowledge is too wonderful for me; it is high, I cannot attain it" (Psalm 139:1-6). Your Father loves you and wants you to be comfortable in His presence. Sometimes we need to learn how to hear His voice and feel His presence, and this is a perfect time to start learning and moving into this special place with your Father.

2. **Plan.** Take some quality time to plan your fast. What is your purpose for the fast? When will it begin for you? When will you complete it, and is there something you will do to acknowledge the finishing point? Review your calendar and consider the appointments and activities that are planned. Do you need to change any of them? Do you need to make special arrangements due to the fast? What study and devotional materials will you need? Do you need to purchase them or order them online? Consider what your day will be like when you are fasting. Will you get up early to spend time in prayer, study, and meditation? This is also the time to consider meal preparation during the Daniel Fast. Will you pack lunches for work or school? Can you dedicate several cooking days during the fasting period to save on meal prep time? Try to imagine your days and plan for them with the fast in mind.

3. **Prepare.** Now that you know the time period of your fast, your purpose, the study materials you want, and ideas about meal planning, this is the step where you actually get busy and get everything ready. I hope you will take the time to read through all the sections in this book so you will be well informed about prayer and fasting before you begin. You will also want to prepare your physical body for the

fast. Ten days before the fast, start drinking at least one half gallon of pure water each day. Taper off caffeine consumption and cut down on sugar and foods that include chemicals. Taking these important steps will help you avoid some of the discomfort that will take place during the first week of your fast. This is the time to invest yourself in good and thorough preparation.

4. Participate. This is it! You are participating in the fast. You might experience several battles during your fast. Your flesh might rebel because you're not giving in to cravings and hunger pangs. Your body might ache with symptoms of withdrawal from sugar and caffeine. You might feel some fatigue in the first week, but more than likely, you will soon feel better than you have in a long while, with increased energy, clearer thinking, and an overall feeling of health and well-being. Be sure to drink plenty of water—at least a half gallon each day. When the flesh rebels, put your spirit in control and stand your ground.

Most important, put your amazing and loving Father in first place on your schedule! If you are not used to spending time with God, ask the Holy Spirit to guide you and teach you. Allow your Father's love to enter your heart. Become familiar with Him. Learn how to live a Spirit-led life and allow Him to work in your life. He is so eager to demonstrate His love for you . . . and He is eager for you to put your hand in His as a child does with a trustworthy and caring Father.

5. Praise and process. Thank God for this experience and all the blessings and lessons He's given you during this period. Spend some time looking back on your experience to process what you learned and think about any permanent changes you may want to make. Very likely, you will have developed some positive and healthy habits that you want to carry forward even though the fast is complete. If you "messed up," consider what you will do next time to reach victory. Review your fast and make notes of those elements that worked well for you and what you will want to change the next time.

Let's look at each of these five steps in greater detail.

PRAY

You are entering this experience to draw closer to the Lord and to hear His direction for your life or the lives of others. Even now, begin praying to your Father and ask Him to bless you. Open your heart to Him so that He will show you truths that He wants you to know. Dedicate yourself and the fast to Him. And listen for His words as you purpose to position yourself humbly before your Lord. This is the most important step as you prepare for your fast.

Several years ago, I heard a Bible teacher talk about making a quality decision to study God's Word every day. The term *quality decision* captured my attention. *Just what is a quality decision?* I wondered. What I have learned since then has helped me immeasurably, and I believe these lessons can make a big difference for you as you approach your Daniel Fast.

A quality decision is one that is firm, deliberate, and entered into with consideration and forethought. When you make a quality decision, you plan to employ the full strength of your will to follow through. A quality decision is when you say, "With God as my guide, Jesus as my strength, and the Holy Spirit as my helper, I am going to do this! I've considered the task. I've measured the effect. And I make the quality decision to complete this commitment."

A quality decision is one in which you fully intend to do your part to fulfill the obligation. For me, a quality decision is a promise to myself and to God that I will do my very best. I won't "wimp out" or step back when the going gets rough. As the Word says, "Therefore put on the full armor of God, so that when the day of evil comes, you may be able to stand your ground, and after you have done everything, to stand" (Ephesians 6:13, NIV). A quality decision means I am fully committed to stand my ground.

Why is this so important? Because it's likely that there will be times when you want to quit or give in a little. You may come home tired and frazzled after a hard day at the office and the last thing you want to eat is another bowl of bean soup or another bite of tofu. Or you'll be home alone, just you and your cravings. Who's going to know if you have one little slice of bread or one little

> " I can already see how preparing the ingredients for the recipes beforehand will help me be successful on the fast.
> —Barbara "

bite of chocolate? Or you get a call from a friend who invites you to lunch at your favorite rib restaurant or steak house. "Just one little lunch," you reason. "I'll just have the petite-cut T-bone, and then I'll get right back on the fast for dinner."

Oh, and then there will be times when the alarm clock buzzes before dawn and you just want to stay nestled under your cozy comforter rather than getting up to study God's Word. Or when your favorite show comes on television and you have to make a choice between watching it or memorizing that verse the Holy Spirit told you to get rooted in your heart. These struggles are an integral part of fasting, but if you've made a quality decision, you can fight through the struggles and you can win. In these times of temptation and weakness, a quality decision will help you to stir up your resolve, seek the Holy Spirit for help, and develop self-control and patience. These are all lessons and exercises that build us up, strengthen us, and provide experiences from which we can draw later in life when the stakes are much higher than a meal or memorizing a Bible verse.

So by making a quality decision, you have made a firm commitment to yourself. To break the firm commitment will require at least the same forethought and consideration. When you are more conscious of your actions, you can actually "watch yourself" as you relinquish power to your flesh. For example, as part of the Daniel Fast, you make a quality decision to not eat bread. But one day you find yourself out shopping, and the local drive-through seems to be calling your name! Your spirit is willing, but your flesh is weak . . . so you turn into the drive-through lane. You know what you are doing, and this gives an opportunity to pause and reconsider your actions. Who is going to win this battle? The spirit or the flesh?

PLAN

You may think this a little strange, but I often call meetings with one person: me! I've labeled them "little meetings with myself," and I actually convene them several times a month. When you prepare for your fast, I strongly encourage you to have a meeting with yourself. Set aside some time when you won't be interrupted and take a look at you. Have a conversation with yourself and look at important things like your goals, your relationships, and your life.

The truth is, so many of us live unintentionally or out of habit or routine. How many times do we say, "Oh, I just wasn't thinking"? We get into schedules and ways of life that form a momentum of their own, and we just go along for the ride. Then we look back and wonder what happened to all the time!

But God said we are fearfully and wonderfully made. We have great minds and powerful imaginations. When they are subject to God, amazing things can happen. We can live conscientiously, with intention and on purpose—His purpose for us! But we must make the choice to take the time to think and make wise decisions for our lives—one day at a time.

James 1:5 tells us, "If any of you lacks wisdom, let him ask of God, who gives to all liberally and without reproach, and it will be given to him."

So call a little meeting with yourself. Take a review of what's going on in your life. This is not a time for condemnation or remorse, but rather a time to take stock of yourself. The Daniel Fast is a perfect time to conduct this self study! Start by clearing your head of thoughts like *I can't do that* or *that's a silly thought*, and instead open your heart to the Holy Spirit and to your own deepest desires. Then get a notebook or tablet and answer the following questions:

- **What five things would you like to accomplish over the next twelve months?** Your answer might include goals like family dinners at least five days each week, learning a new hobby, memorizing one Bible verse each week, traveling to a place where you've longed to go, attending a Christian conference, or working toward a promotion at work. Let the goals come from within you. If you are like most people, there are many unrealized dreams and desires in your heart.

- **What are three new habits you want to form?** Do you want to establish a morning routine that enables you to meet with your Father each day for at least one hour? Do you want to lose that extra weight once and for all? Do you want to watch television less and read more? Do you want to make a habit of complimenting your spouse and children three times each day? Again, tap into those unrealized hopes in your heart.

- **What fears do you have that you want God to help you conquer?** Do you have the fear of not having enough money when you reach retirement? Are you afraid of people and their opinions of you? Are you afraid the economy will get so bad that you will not have enough to care for your needs?

- **Is there unforgiveness in your heart?** If you answered no to that question, then bless you! I can say that because so many of us have unresolved hurts and unforgiven wrongs that still weigh on us. Perhaps even while you read these words, some thoughts or memories are bubbling to the surface.

- **Are there areas that are "out of order" in your life?** Are there projects that are looming over your head or personal challenges that you need to tackle? Is there a relationship that needs your attention or an item on your "I really need to get that done" list that continues to nag at you? List a few items that are out of order so you can address them.

Consider your list and select one or two goals as your focus for prayer, study, and action during your Daniel Fast. This will be your purpose for your fast.

A few years ago, I made a decision that I wanted to rid myself of some unforgiveness that lingered in my heart. I had tried to forgive this person many times before, but wasn't successful. I realized that I really didn't know how to forgive when a great wrong had been done to me! I needed help. So I focused my Daniel Fast on learning about forgiveness and doing the work of forgiving this person. I purchased a copy of *Total Forgiveness* by R. T. Kendall. Each evening I read a chapter of the book, and then during my morning quiet time with the Lord, I talked to Him about what I was learning and shared my thoughts, hurts, and desire to forgive with Him.

The Holy Spirit guided me through this process and taught me how to replace hurtful memories with prayers of thanksgiving. Kendall's book helped me understand what forgiveness is about and guided me through the process of fully forgiving this person. Every once in a while, a sad memory will pop up, but now I am equipped to "take that thought into captivity" and replace it with a good thought and a short prayer.

Our Father wants us to examine ourselves so we can become the strong and healthy individuals He knows we can be! We are called to this duty of self-examination: "For if we would judge ourselves, we would not be judged. But when we are judged, we are chastened by the Lord, that we may not be condemned with the world" (1 Corinthians 11:31-32). The term *chastened* means "to instruct for learning." When we look at our shortcomings, our loving Father will show us what we need to do to change from weakness to strength. And if we spend the time to take a close look inside, we can learn new ways before we fall and have to pick up the broken and cracked pieces.

As you plan for your fast, be sure to schedule a consistent time to meet with the Lord. Starting the day with quiet time seems to work the best for many people. There are fewer chances of interruptions or delays, and it's also a perfect foundation for the day. But if your situation doesn't allow for the morning, then select a time that is good for you. The key is consistency. Daniel was a very busy man with all his duties and responsibilities and he was living in a foreign land that had different customs and worshiped false gods. But Daniel still maintained the Jewish practice of morning, midday, and evening prayer. This daily feeding of the spirit enables God to interact with you and the Word of God to guide and direct you.

So as you plan your fast, be sure to set aside a daily time when you can be one-on-one with the Lord.

Plan how you will pray, meditate, and study during your fast

Perhaps you are a mature Christian and have developed habits that support your spiritual growth and relationship with God. If you've found practices that work for you, then great! This section is to help those who are still struggling in their prayer life and haven't yet found a blueprint that meets their needs. If that's you, please know that you are not alone. I hear from hundreds of men and women who struggle in this area.

There are many ways to approach Bible study, prayer, and meditation, and the Daniel Fast is a perfect opportunity to develop good habits and spiritual disciplines. As you plan for your fast, you'll want to consider exactly how and what you will study during this time. I will share some methods that have worked for me and others, but please understand this list is not exhaustive. I encourage you to try some patterns and find a routine that works for you. Remember, the most important thing is that you want to develop a discipline that will draw you into a personal, deep, and abiding relationship with your Father.

That being said, however, let me share one essential key to growing in your relationship with God: consistency. I'm not talking about legalism, where you fail if you don't start praying each day at 6:00 a.m. or if you read four chapters from the Bible instead of five. This kind of thinking focuses on the activity rather than on the result you want to achieve, which in this case is a growing and intimate relationship with your Father.

Spiritual legalism is very different from a spiritual discipline. In this context, a discipline is a habit or routine that is consistently practiced for a specific purpose. Our Christian faith employs many spiritual disciplines, including prayer, fasting, tithing, Bible study, and service. I like to think of spiritual disciplines as behaviors in Kingdom living. When we follow the commandments of God, we are exercising our spiritual disciplines.

> I have found this way of eating so beneficial that for the first time in ages I feel that eating chocolate is not worth the fatigue it causes afterward.
>
> —Charlotte

Jesus had many spiritual disciplines. In Luke 4:16 we read of one: "So He came to Nazareth, where He had been brought up. And as His custom was, He went into the synagogue on the Sabbath day, and stood up to read." The words "as His custom was" tell us that going to the synagogue on the Sabbath was His routine, His habit, His spiritual discipline. Throughout the New Testament we can see how Jesus practiced many consistent habits that kept Him close to the Father.

So in order to be successful, we want to develop spiritual disciplines that we can practice consistently. As followers of Christ, we want these disciplines to align with the Word of God and the teachings of Jesus. Following Christ's model will keep us within the limits of our faith, build toward our success, help us to hear from God, and guard us from making mistakes. Plan ahead for your success and move to intentionally pursue your Father. The rewards are greater than you can imagine. They are not the rewards of this world. They are much better! They are the rewards of the Kingdom of God!

Establish a time and place

First, define a time when you can have one-on-one time with God where interruptions and distractions are minimized. For most people, this is early morning. My pastor, David Saltzman, practices what I call "Crest and Christ." Every morning he wakes up, brushes his teeth, and then spends time with God. He doesn't wake up at the same time every day. Some days he may sleep a little later. But when he does wake up, he does the same thing. He brushes his teeth, and before getting distracted with any other activity, he spends time with God. When the rare occasion arises when he can't follow this discipline, he says he feels out of sorts and is eager to return to the routine the next day.

My routine is also in the mornings. When I'm not fasting I have what I call "coffee with Jesus." As soon as I get up, I make a piping hot cup of coffee (I've spent most of my life in Seattle—the hometown for Starbucks—where coffee is almost a cultural obligation). Then I go back to my cozy bed, position my pillows, and say, "Good morning, Lord." That's the start to my great time with God. When I fast, I replace the coffee with a cup of hot water with lemon.

Usually I start by telling Him how much I love Him and that I am so thankful for His love and care for me. I don't make these statements religiously. The truth is, I am regularly staggered and humbled by God's great care for me. So it's not difficult to genuinely thank and praise Him for His goodness, love, and provision.

Then the routine part of my time with God leaves, because I don't do the same thing every day. Sometimes I will read the Bible and then stop and meditate on a verse or passage that's caught my heart. I might read from a Christian book or magazine, usually about a subject that links to something I'm working on to build my faith. There are times when I ask the Holy Spirit very specific questions about things I don't understand, or I ask Him to help me with a weakness in myself or a situation in my life.

I consistently spend at least an hour doing this every day, though many times I find two or three hours have passed before I'm ready to get on with my day! Granted, I am in a unique situation since my children are grown and I work from my home. But when my children were younger, I still spent just about every morning having coffee with Jesus. It's a habit that has blessed me over the years.

So as you plan for your fast, I do encourage you to define a time when you can be with God. Don't think about developing a habit that will last for the rest of your life. Instead, mull over what you can do during this period of fasting. Set yourself up for success! If an hour seems impossible for you right now, then have a little meeting with yourself and consider what could work for you. Can you start with thirty minutes? Do mornings feel impossible for you? Perhaps evenings are better for you and your lifestyle. The key is to define a time and place where you can be alone with God on a consistent and daily basis.

Decide on a method to get into the Word of God

There are so many ways to study the Bible. I've used many approaches over the years, and often the way I study has a lot to do with what's going on in my spiritual life at the time. We've already talked about defining your purpose for fasting. This purpose will likely guide the approach you take to digging into God's Word.

Generally when I fast, I create a study plan. For example, several years ago I wanted to learn how to pray more effectively. The Word says, "Therefore I say to you, whatever things you ask when you pray, believe that you receive them, and you will have them" (Mark 11:24). But that had not been my experience. There were a lot of times when I prayed but didn't receive what I asked for. I believe the Bible to be true, and I knew God wasn't failing. So I decided to focus on effective prayer during my fast. I bought a couple of books about how to pray. One was a workbook, so I put together a notebook where I could write out my answers. I also compiled a list of Scriptures concerning prayer. Then, on my first day of the fast, I asked the Holy Spirit to help me learn to pray effectively.

Each day I learned what the Bible had to say about prayer. I learned of some mistakes I was making in the way I was praying, and I started forming new habits. As I studied the verses in the Bible, I tried to imagine the scene with me in it. I read the footnotes in my Bible concerning each verse, and I looked up the Hebrew and Greek meanings of some of the words. I learned about the various kinds of prayer and how to match the type of prayer with the need. I talked to God about what I was learning, and I started to pray using my new knowledge and understanding. I could feel my faith building as I learned more about the awesome nature of God when I read books, prayed, meditated, and utilized Bible reference tools.

This study launched me into a new and greater understanding of God, our relationship to Him, and our position in the world as children of the Most High King. These morning times were rich and rewarding and lifted me to a new level in my faith.

Mine for nuggets

When my friend Ron Jackson reads through one of the books of the Bible, he tries to find one nugget of truth in each chapter. When he completes the chapter he takes a few minutes to think back on what he's just read. When he's captured the nugget in his mind, he thinks about how it links with the rest of the book. This simple method has helped Ron not only to grow in faith as he learns about the ways of God, but also to remember where certain passages are in the Bible. I recently used this method while studying the book of Romans and found it to be very helpful. When I paused to identify the specific nugget of each chapter, I also prayed and talked to God about what I was learning.

Do some weeding

Another way to study the Word of God is to let it be our teacher to mold us and shape us into the image of Christ. For example, take a few minutes and read Mark 4:1-20. Read the words aloud. Picture yourself sitting on the grassy field by the sea. Try to imagine Jesus speaking directly to you as He teaches about the sower and the seed. Listen with your heart open for insight.

Now, consider the condition of your heart. How is your heart compared to the four described in the parable? Are there some weeds that need pulling? Is there some cultivating that needs to take place? Does your ground need some care so that the Word of God can take hold, grow, and bear fruit?

This is just one example of how you can use the Scriptures to change your life! It's a powerful and living Word and ready to reveal God's truths to us.

Study a word

I love this method of digging into the Word of God. Again, depending on the purpose of your fast, think of a word—for example, *faith*. Then use a concordance, or one of the many online tools available, and look up each verse that includes that word. I like finding the verses in my own Bible. There's something about reading the verses in my own personal Bible that helps me in subsequent studies. I sometimes make notes or underline the verses. I like to mark up my Bible. I write comments and mark verses that strike my spirit when I'm studying. I have a small plastic box that's packed with markers and gel pens. I also have little Post-it Notes to mark pages. Using these tools helps me in my study and recall.

Get to know Jesus

This is one of my favorite ways to explore the Word of God because it changed my life forever! I am a baby boomer whose teen and early adult years were influenced by the sixties and seventies in Seattle, a city known for its independent thinking. I wasn't a Christian then, and like many who grew up in that era, I questioned the status quo and didn't accept beliefs just because of tradition or cultural conventions.

One morning in 1973 (I was in my early twenties at the time), I answered a knock at my door and found two women toting their Bibles and religious literature. They introduced themselves and asked if I believed in the Bible. I said I thought it was a good book with a lot of good stories. Then they asked me if I believed Jesus was the Son of God, to which my response was, "Well, I think Jesus was a good teacher and a good man. But I don't think He's really the Son of God."

Their next question sparked a need for a quick answer from me: "Would you like to learn more about Jesus? We would be happy to share with you." I didn't believe Jesus was anything more than a wise man, but I wasn't prepared to debate them. I needed more time.

"Well," I said, fumbling for words so I sounded like I was in control, "I can't meet with you right now. But how about if you come back next week and we can talk then?" They agreed, and we said our good-byes. As I shut the door, I thought to myself, *I'm going to be ready for you gals. I'll show you.*

I needed to learn fast, because I didn't know a lot about the Bible. I found a copy in some packed-away books I had and started my cram sessions. Each night before I went to sleep, I read the Bible so I could learn about this guy, Jesus. I started with the Gospel of Matthew and continued until my eyes were heavy and it was time to sleep. I did this for several nights.

I don't remember where I was reading, but I do recall the sensation that went through my soul when I suddenly rested the book on my chest, looked out into the room, and said, "Oh God, this is true!" Like in the hymn, "Amazing Grace," that was the moment "I first believed." The powerful Living Word of God penetrated my soul, and at that moment the truth captured me forever. My spirit was born again, and I went to sleep that night as a new creature in Christ.

The next day I visited my neighbor who for several months had gently witnessed to me, answering questions and being an example of a Christ-centered woman. I told her what had happened to me, and she invited me to attend church with her the next Sunday. I went along, and a few weeks later made my public confession that Christ was my Lord.

I never saw the two women who had started the "learn about Jesus" ball in motion. But from that momentous night, I have forever been changed. For that I am eternally thankful.

So reading the Bible to learn about Jesus is special to me. And I still occasionally approach the Gospels in this way. I'll slowly and thoughtfully read a passage and then try to picture the scene in my mind. I try to imagine Jesus, the expression on His face when He speaks, and His mood. I do the same with the others in the scene, whether they are disciples, Pharisees, or someone else. Then I place myself in the scene and try to hear Jesus speaking the words so they can enter into my heart and work in my spirit. Sometimes I'll stop and talk to the Lord about what I'm learning or ask questions if there is something I don't quite get. This is a powerful way to study the Word of God and get to know Christ in an intimate way.

Study a book in the Bible

The Bible contains sixty-six different books, each filled with various truths about God, testimonies of men and women and how their faith impacted their lives and situations, and lessons for us to learn so we can live Christ-centered and holy lives. I have been studying the Word of God for more than thirty-five years now, and I am still amazed at the abundance of truth it contains. The more I learn, the more I am stunned by the intricate ways in which the precepts all link together. The power in the living Word of God is another one of the mysteries that only those who are alive in the Spirit can grasp.

We are so blessed to have a profusion of study materials to help us grow in the knowledge and love of Christ. Using a commentary and a study guide to dig into a specific book in the Bible can be an enriching practice. First, decide what book you want to study. Ask the Holy Spirit to guide you in your selection, and within a day or two, if your spiritual eyes and ears are open, you will receive His direction. Then find a study guide by visiting your local bookstore or searching online.

I consider the book of Daniel an excellent choice to study during the Daniel Fast. I like to focus on the character qualities of the prophet and his companions and how they lived out their faith for decades while in captivity in a hostile and godless culture.

You also may want to read "the Proverb for the day." There are thirty-one chapters in the book of Proverbs, so match the chapter number with the date and you're ready to go! For example, if it's the fifth day of the month, read Proverbs 5. Easy and simple. You can also add Psalms to your monthly reading routine if you'd like by reading five psalms each day. Multiply the date times five each day to find which psalm to start with. For example, if it's the fifth day of the month, multiply five by five. You would then read Psalms 25–29 for the day. This method is a powerful way to feed your spirit with God's love and truth.

Find your true identity

As Christians we are sure about being heaven bound, but many who profess Christ as their Savior don't realize that we are also the fully adopted and completely righteous children of the Most High God. For the better part of my Christian life, I missed out on many benefits of my inheritance because I didn't really know who I was in Christ. Oh, I knew I was a Christian and that I was going to heaven, but until I started digging into the Word of God and finding my birthright, I was living the life of a waif—even though the Kingdom of God was fully available to me.

I'm still learning how to fully live as an heir to the throne. But today my life is full, rich, and abundant because I am a joint heir with Christ. How about you? When you think of yourself as a joint heir with Christ, does your heart leap with joy? Or do you shrink back and think to yourself, *I know the Bible says that, but I really don't believe it.*

My son is adopted, and to make it legal, the United States

government issued official papers giving him full rights as a member of our family. In a similar way, the Bible, the Word of God, serves as official adoption papers for everyone who is born again of the Spirit. Romans 8:15-17 states this:

> *For you did not receive the spirit of bondage again to fear, but you received the Spirit of adoption by whom we cry out, "Abba, Father." The Spirit Himself bears witness with our spirit that we are children of God, and if children, then heirs—heirs of God and joint heirs with Christ, if indeed we suffer with Him, that we may also be glorified together.*

Because of Christ, we are adopted. And just like Christ, we can cry out with the familiar and loving salutation of "Abba, Father." We are joint heirs with Jesus. I know that's a lot to swallow. I'm still getting it! But if you can lay hold of the truth of who you are because of Christ, your self-esteem issues will begin to disappear and your confidence will begin to rise. It won't be a prideful confidence, but rather an unshakable sense that Christ is alive in you and you are a precious child of God. It's a confidence in your God like that of Daniel in the den of lions.

To help discover your true identity in the Scriptures, use a concordance and search out New Testament verses that include these words and phrases:

- in Him
- through Him
- with Him
- in Christ
- through Christ
- with Christ
- in Jesus
- through Jesus
- with Jesus

Once you find these verses, think about each one and—even though your mind (which has been conditioned by the god of this world) might be fighting you all the way—start telling yourself that these words are describing you! Here are just a few of the hundreds of verses you can find:

Likewise you also, reckon yourselves to be dead indeed to sin, but alive to God in Christ Jesus *our Lord.*
—ROMANS 6:11, EMPHASIS ADDED

For the wages of sin is death, but the gift of God is eternal life *in Christ Jesus our Lord.* —ROMANS 6:23, EMPHASIS ADDED

There is therefore now no condemnation to those who are in Christ Jesus, *who do not walk according to the flesh, but according to the Spirit.* —ROMANS 8:1, EMPHASIS ADDED

For the law of the Spirit of life in Christ Jesus has made me free from the law of sin and death. —ROMANS 8:2

Yet in all these things we are more than conquerors through Him *who loved us.* —ROMANS 8:37, EMPHASIS ADDED

For I am persuaded that neither death nor life, nor angels nor principalities nor powers, nor things present nor things to come, nor height nor depth, nor any other created thing, shall be able to separate us from the love of God which is in Christ Jesus *our Lord.* —ROMANS 8:38-39, EMPHASIS ADDED

If we endure, we shall also reign with Him. *If we deny Him, He also will deny us.* —2 TIMOTHY 2:12, EMPHASIS ADDED

Coming to Him as to a living stone, rejected indeed by men, but chosen by God and precious, you also, as living stones, are being built up a spiritual house, a holy priesthood, to offer up spiritual sacrifices acceptable to God through Jesus Christ. —1 PETER 2:4-5

Remember, your fast is a spiritual discipline. It's easy to focus so much on the change in diet that the prayer and meditation can fall behind. So again, plan for your successful fast by choosing the methods you will use to consistently feed on God's Word. You will be pleased if you take time to plan the spiritual food you will feed your spirit during your Daniel Fast. Remember what Jesus said: "It is written, 'Man shall not live by bread alone, but by every word that proceeds from the mouth of God'" (Matthew 4:4).

Determine what you will and will not eat during the Daniel Fast

As we already established, fasting is always about restricting food for a spiritual purpose. We've already talked about establishing a purpose for your fast. But now I would like to direct your focus onto your physical body, which is certainly engaged during the Daniel Fast.

Your Creator formed you. Whether you're pleased with your body right now or not, you are fearfully and wonderfully made. All of creation, including your human body, is the masterpiece of our Father. And He created everything to work together for good. He designed our physical bodies with marvelous systems to sustain life and give us the energy we need to function. He produced food to fuel us and organs within our bodies to consume, digest, and then distribute the nourishment. During the Daniel Fast, we don't use any processed foods because they have had the life and goodness stripped from them. We want to feed our bodies with the foods our Creator designed especially for us.

As you plan for your Daniel Fast, take some time to consider what you will eat and what you will drink. Think about your physical body and its condition. This could be a wonderful time of renewal and adopting healthy habits.

Let's take a walk back into our high school health science class. This information will help you understand some important facts about your body and give you tools for a successful Daniel Fast.

When we eat food, our bodies secrete digestive enzymes to break down the food into simpler components. These elements then move into the cells that line our digestive tract so the nutrients can travel into the bloodstream for distribution throughout the body to meet the needs of life.

Each time we consume food, we take in not only the good nutrients that our bodies need, but also additives and toxins that may be hitchhiking in the foods. God designed our amazing bodies so that the elements that are not suitable for health are filtered out by the digestive tract, the liver, the kidneys, and other organs. This process also takes away non-nutrient matter, such as by-products of digestion, bacterial waste from the decomposition of inadequately digested foodstuffs, and excess nutrients the body can't use. So our physical systems work hard to remove what is not useful. To make things worse for our bodies, when we eat foods loaded with chemicals and toxins, overeat, and don't chew our foods properly, we are taxing our digestive systems even more.

We've all experienced times when our digestive systems have been overworked. That's when we face the gurgling stomach, the bloated belly, or the "why did I eat the whole thing" blues. Our bodies are telling us to take better care of them.

The truth is that our bodies can take a lot of abuse before they begin to scream for our attention. At first, it might be a few aches and pains, or we might feel a little tired. Perhaps we're not able to ward off illnesses as quickly. Eventually, however, the screaming continues until it finally gets so loud that we have to listen. The scale can certainly tell us a thing or two when a shocking number registers! The doctor may serve as the translator when he or she says, "The tests are back and you have diabetes" or "You have an autoimmune disease that's causing all that pain in your joints." Hopefully the warning doesn't come from an emergency medical technician shouting to everybody in the room, "All clear!" as electrical paddles reboot our hearts.

According to the Trust for America's Health, which examines

obesity trends and policies each year, U. S. adult obesity is climbing at an alarming rate. In a 2008 report entitled *F as in Fat: How
Obesity Policies Are Failing in America,* the group documented that
the rate increased in thirty-seven states in 2007. Not one state saw
a decrease. In addition to the serious health impacts associated
with obesity—type 2 diabetes rates rose in twenty-six states—the
Department of Health and Human Services reports that obese
and overweight adults cost the United States anywhere from $69
billion to $117 billion per year. The current rise in food prices,
coupled with the economic recession, raises serious concerns about
obesity, as the high cost of many healthful foods can be prohibi-
tive for some Americans. In fact, nutritionists are now worried
that Americans will put on "recession pounds," pointing to studies linking obesity and unhealthy eating habits to low incomes.[5]

Too many of us are not taking care of the bodies God so
beautifully created. According to the Centers for Disease Control and Prevention (CDC), the rate of new cases of diagnosed
diabetes rose by more than 90 percent among adults over the last
ten years. This and other studies indicate that about 8 percent of
the American population now has diabetes, mainly type 2 diabetes, which is linked to obesity and sedentary living. One quarter
of people aged sixty and older have diabetes. The World Health
Organization (WHO) calls this disease an epidemic, estimating
that the number of people worldwide with diabetes will double
to 366 million by 2030. Most people with diabetes have resistance to insulin, which the body uses to convert blood sugar to
energy.[6]

The prevalence of obesity in the United States continues to be
a health concern for adults, children, and adolescents. Recent sur-
veys show that more than 33 percent of adult men and more than
35 percent of adult women are obese. The younger generations
seem to be well on their way to the same outcome, with more than
16 percent of children and adolescents tipping the scales to obesity. This rate of obesity raises concern because of its implications

for the health of Americans. Obesity increases the risk of many diseases and health conditions. These include the following:

- coronary heart disease
- type 2 diabetes
- cancers (endometrial, breast, and colon)
- hypertension (high blood pressure)
- dyslipidemia (for example, high total cholesterol or high levels of triglycerides)
- stroke
- liver and gallbladder disease
- sleep apnea and respiratory problems
- osteoarthritis (a degeneration of cartilage and its underlying bone within a joint)
- gynecological problems (abnormal menses, infertility)

These are just some of the health factors and consequences of not taking care of our bodies. And that's why I believe the growing popularity of the Daniel Fast among God's children is so timely. We have an opportunity to enter a period of prayer and fasting in which we present our whole selves to God. A significant part of this act of submission is to adhere to the boundaries of eating foods that are good for us and that are designed by our Creator to nourish our bodies.

Digestion

Let's look at the digestive system, which starts in your mouth when you chew your food. The food then passes through the esophagus and into the stomach, where strong muscles churn and mash the food into smaller and smaller pieces with help from gastric juices that come from the stomach's walls. In addition to breaking down food, gastric juices also help kill bacteria that might be in the food.

The food then passes to the small intestine, which is a long and narrow tube that is about twenty-three feet long in adults. Its function is to break down the food even more and extract the vitamins, minerals, proteins, carbohydrates, and fats. This is where the pancreas and kidneys come in as they contribute their digestive juices to the process. The pancreatic juices help the body digest fats and protein. Bile comes from the liver; it emulsifies fats and neutralizes acids in food so they can be absorbed into the bloodstream. The gallbladder serves as a storage unit for extra bile. During this storage time, the bile becomes more concentrated than when it left the liver and its potency is increased, thus intensifying its effect on fats when the body needs it.

Food stays in the small intestine many hours so that the nutrients can pass from the organ to the bloodstream. The nutrient-rich blood flows directly to the liver, which filters out harmful substances and wastes. The liver also helps control what nutrients will go to the rest of the body and what will stay behind in storage. For example, the liver stores certain vitamins and a type of sugar the body uses for energy. All food not digested through these processes is then passed on to the large intestine.

The large intestine is so called because it is wide in diameter; however, it is actually shorter than the small intestine, only about five feet long (1.5 meters).[7] Add the two intestines together, and that's a whopping twenty-eight feet of tubing through which the food we eat must pass! When the waste reaches this station in the digestive process, the large intestine—also called the colon—has one more chance to absorb water or minerals into the blood. This final stage is where most of the liquid is removed, and the remaining substance is the stool.

Fiber

It only takes a little research about healthy diets to discover two things: (1) our bodies need a lot of fiber for good health, and (2) the reason so many people experience improved health while on the Daniel Fast is the extra fiber they eat while on it.

Dietary fiber, sometimes called roughage, is the indigestible portion of plant foods that pushes matter through the small and large intestine, absorbing water and easing elimination. Dietary fiber is found mainly in fruits, vegetables, whole grains, and legumes. It's probably best known for its ability to prevent or relieve constipation. However, fiber can provide other health benefits as well, such as lowering your risk of diabetes and heart disease. Fiber is essential to help food move through the digestive system quickly.

Here's what the Mayo Clinic reports about fiber:

Dietary fiber, also known as roughage or bulk, includes all parts of plant foods that your body can't digest or absorb. Unlike other food components such as fats, proteins, or carbohydrates—which your body breaks down and absorbs— fiber isn't digested by your body. Therefore, it passes virtually unchanged through your stomach and small intestine and into your colon.

Fiber is often classified into two categories: those that don't dissolve in water (insoluble fiber) and those that do (soluble fiber).

- Insoluble fiber. This type of fiber promotes the movement of material through your digestive system and increases stool bulk, so it can benefit those who struggle with constipation or irregular stools. Whole wheat flour, wheat bran, nuts, and many vegetables are good sources of insoluble fiber.
- Soluble fiber. This type of fiber dissolves in water to form a gel-like material. It can help lower blood cholesterol and glucose levels. You can find generous quantities of soluble fiber in oats, peas, beans, apples, citrus fruits, carrots, barley, and psyllium.

The amount of each type of fiber varies in different plant foods. To receive the greatest health benefit, eat a wide variety of high-fiber foods.[8]

As you plan the foods you will eat during your Daniel Fast, take a look at the fiber content of some common foods. Read nutrition labels to find out exactly how much fiber is in your favorite foods. Recommended fiber amounts are 21 to 25 grams a day for women and 30 to 38 grams a day for men. All foods on the following list are acceptable on the Daniel Fast.

FIBER CONTENT OF COMMON FOODS*

Fruits	Serving Size	Total Fiber (grams)
Raspberries	1 cup	8.0
Pear, with skin	1 medium	5.1
Apple, with skin	1 medium	4.4
Figs, dried	2 medium	3.7
Blueberries	1 cup	3.5
Strawberries	1 cup	3.3
Banana	1 medium	3.1
Orange	1 medium	3.1
Raisins	1.5 ounce box	1.6
Grains, Cereal, and Pasta	Serving Size	Total Fiber (grams)
Spaghetti, whole wheat, cooked	1 cup	6.3
Barley, pearled, cooked	1 cup	6.0
Wheat bran flakes	¾ cup	5.1
Oatmeal, quick, regular, or instant, cooked	1 cup	4.0
Popcorn, air popped	3 cups	3.6
Brown rice, cooked	1 cup	3.5
Unleavened bread, whole wheat or multigrain	1 slice	1.9

Protein

The typical American diet is very rich in proteins. The fact is that most people consume much more than is necessary, eating meat and/or dairy products with every meal. However, on the Daniel Fast, neither meat nor dairy products are allowed, so we need to look at alternative sources of protein.

Legumes, Nuts, and Seeds	Serving Size	Total Fiber (grams)
Split peas, cooked	1 cup	16.3
Lentils, cooked	1 cup	15.6
Black beans, cooked	1 cup	15.0
Lima beans, cooked	1 cup	13.2
Sunflower seeds, hulled	¼ cup	3.6
Almonds	1 ounce (22 nuts)	3.3
Pistachio nuts	1 ounce (49 nuts)	2.9
Pecans	1 ounce (19 halves)	2.7
Vegetables	Serving Size	Total Fiber (grams)
Artichoke, cooked	1 medium	10.3
Peas, cooked	1 cup	8.8
Broccoli, boiled	1 cup	5.1
Turnip greens, boiled	1 cup	5.0
Sweet corn, cooked	1 cup	4.6
Brussels sprouts, cooked	1 cup	4.1
Potato, with skin, baked	1 medium	4.0
Tomato paste	¼ cup	2.7
Carrot, raw	1 medium	1.7

*Fiber content can vary between brands.[9]

According to the U.S. Food and Drug Administration, the average adult should consume 50 grams of protein each day (based on 2,000 calories a day for adults and children over four). Many health professionals disagree and say we consume far too much protein.

A six-ounce broiled porterhouse steak is a great source of protein—38 grams. But it also delivers 44 grams of fat, 16 of them saturated. That's almost three-fourths of the recommended daily intake for saturated fat. The same amount of salmon gives you 34 grams of protein and 18 grams of fat, 4 of them saturated. A cup of cooked lentils has 18 grams of protein, but less than 1 gram of fat. No wonder people usually lose ten to twenty-five pounds on the Daniel Fast! It's a very low-fat diet.

So when choosing protein-rich foods, pay attention to what comes along with the protein. Vegetable sources of protein, such as beans, nuts, and whole grains as well as tofu and soybeans, are excellent choices, and they offer healthy fiber, vitamins, and minerals.

Water

In Daniel 1, we read that the prophet and his companions drank only water. So that's why the only acceptable beverage on the Daniel Fast is good old H_2O. For many people (including me) this is the most difficult part about the fast. I've enjoyed my morning java for more than forty years, so giving up my daily cup of steaming hot, freshly ground Starbucks dark roast with organic half-and-half is challenging. I do it, but I confess that I really miss my morning coffee when I fast.

Others have a hard time giving up tea and soda. I've heard from many men and women who say they felt addicted to these beverages, and that the Daniel Fast reintroduced them to water. And I can't count the number of times I've had to explain to people that tea is not allowed on the fast. The common argument is, "Well if it's an all-plant diet, and herbal tea is a plant, then why can't I have tea? It's just putting plants in water." It is, however, permissible to add a little lemon juice, fresh mint, or slices of lemon or cucumber to your water, as long as you don't "cross the line" to tea or lemonade.

My customary answer is, "I feel your pain, dear one. But tea is not water; it's tea. And the only beverage on the Daniel Fast is water. See Daniel chapter 1."

I really do feel their pain. I still have to push myself to drink water. But I do it, because I am fully convinced that it's good for my body. The truth is, when we drink adequate water to meet our physical needs, we're taking good care of ourselves. Water is your body's most necessary chemical component and makes up about 60 percent of your body weight. Every system in your body depends on water. Water flushes toxins out of vital organs; it carries nutrients to your cells and provides a moist environment for tissues, including your ears, nose, and throat.[10]

Not drinking enough water can lead to dehydration so that our systems don't have enough water to carry out normal functions. Dehydration can drain your energy and make you tired—plus the message your brain sends for dehydration is often wrongly received as hunger. So we eat when instead we should have satisfied this need with a glass of fresh water.

Consider how you care for God's temple, your body

It's easy to see why we need to make good decisions about what will go into our mouths as food. We have a masterfully designed system to keep us healthy and full of energy. And we can either cooperate with the system—or not.

The Daniel Fast helped me take an honest look at how I was caring for the temple God had entrusted to me. Are you willing to take a look at how you are caring for your body? As you plan for your Daniel Fast, consider the fact that your physical body is either controlled by the Holy Spirit or it's controlled by your flesh. The unreformed soul is the producer of unhealthy cravings, overeating, and emotional eating—also known as "food therapy." God's plan for us, His children, is that we live Kingdom of God lives! Not lives where we are sick, broken, and helpless.

His Word is clear: we are to be in good health and finish strong, living in victory all the days of our lives. In 3 John 1:2 we read, "Beloved, I pray that you may prosper in all things and be in health, just as your soul prospers." Jeremiah 29:11 says, "For I know the thoughts that I think toward you, says the LORD, thoughts of peace and not of evil, to give you a future and a hope."

And why can we have this victorious future? Not because we are so great in ourselves, but because with Christ in us nothing is impossible. Jesus said, "These things I have spoken to you, that in Me you may have peace. In the world you will have tribulation; but be of good cheer, I have overcome the world" (John 16:33). Yes, in Him we can have peace, which means nothing missing and nothing broken. But we must cooperate! The choice is ours.

Consider the powerful truth in this verse:

> *Or do you not know that your body is the temple of the Holy Spirit who is in you, whom you have from God, and you are not your own? For you were bought at a price; therefore glorify God in your body and in your spirit, which are God's.*
>
> —1 CORINTHIANS 6:19-20

The Daniel Fast is a short period of time compared to all the days in this year. God created fasting so His children can draw closer to Him, because He so desperately wants to draw close to us. And the Daniel Fast truly is an occasion when you can feed your soul, strengthen your spirit, and renew your body.

PREPARE
The more we learn about health and nutrition, the better we understand what we should and should not be consuming for the best care of our physical bodies. As you prepare for your fast by planning out your first week of meals, a food pyramid can help you make wise choices.

THE daniel fast food pyramid

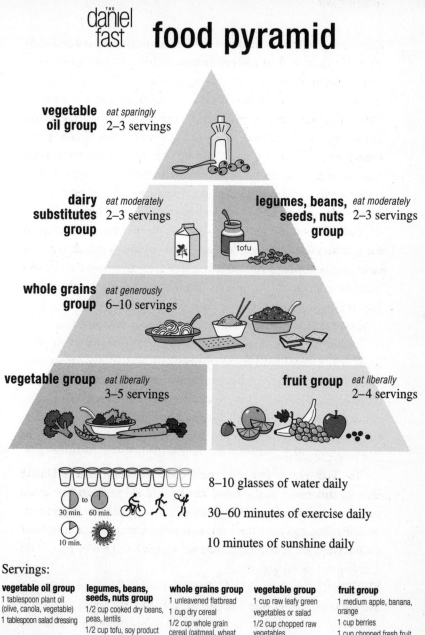

vegetable oil group *eat sparingly* 2–3 servings

dairy substitutes group *eat moderately* 2–3 servings

legumes, beans, seeds, nuts group *eat moderately* 2–3 servings

whole grains group *eat generously* 6–10 servings

vegetable group *eat liberally* 3–5 servings

fruit group *eat liberally* 2–4 servings

8–10 glasses of water daily

30 min. to 60 min. — 30–60 minutes of exercise daily

10 min. — 10 minutes of sunshine daily

Servings:

vegetable oil group
1 tablespoon plant oil (olive, canola, vegetable)
1 tablespoon salad dressing

dairy substitutes group
1 cup soy, rice, or almond milk used in recipes

legumes, beans, seeds, nuts group
1/2 cup cooked dry beans, peas, lentils
1/2 cup tofu, soy product
2 tablespoons nut butter
1/4 cup nuts

whole grains group
1 unleavened flatbread
1 cup dry cereal
1/2 cup whole grain cereal (oatmeal, wheat flakes, muesli)
1/2 cup cooked rice
1/2 cup whole wheat pasta
3–4 whole grain crackers

vegetable group
1 cup raw leafy green vegetables or salad
1/2 cup chopped raw vegetables
1/2 cup cooked vegetables

fruit group
1 medium apple, banana, orange
1 cup berries
1 cup chopped fresh fruit
3/4 cup dried fruit

This food pyramid is intended for a temporary partial-fast eating plan. Consult your health professional whenever you make a significant change in your eating and/or exercise habits.

Choose the foods you will eat ahead of time. Since so many of today's prepared food items include highly processed ingredients, chemicals, and sweeteners, you will likely make most of your meals from scratch. If you are not accustomed to preparing recipes from scratch, you might feel a little overwhelmed at this point and be asking yourself, *How in the world can I prepare all these meals, work a full-time job, take care of my family, and still have time for God?*

I understand the quandary. I have a special place in my heart for mothers who try their best to juggle all the demands on their time and attention. Still, there is a way for you to not only have a good experience with your own Daniel Fast, but also support your family in good eating habits. Plus, you might even develop some habits and systems that assist you beyond your fasting days.

I spent many years working as a consultant to Christian organizations. A common business principle I advised was "Plan your work. Work your plan," because it's often an essential ingredient for efficiency, effectiveness, and wise financial stewardship. The principle also works in the home, and certainly with meal preparation. A small investment of preparation before the fast even begins can reap great benefits.

You will find it easier to make food decisions for the Daniel Fast if you lock on to these details: the Daniel Fast is a plant-based eating plan with additional restrictions that include no sweeteners, no leavening products, and no man-made chemicals or processed foods. For a more complete outline, review the Daniel Fast Food List beginning on page 99.

Engaging the practice of "Plan your work. Work your plan" is as easy as following these simple steps:

1. **Create menus, along with your shopping list, for the coming week.** Use the Daniel Fast recipes to plan

your daily menus, check ingredients you have on hand, review store ads for sales, and clip coupons or download them from the Internet. You can search a manufacturer's website to find coupons for the company's products that are redeemable at your local store. You are now equipped to shop. Also, consider activities that may be on your calendar and school or work lunches that need to be prepared when planning the week's menus. Try to make only one weekly shopping trip.

2. **Prepare ingredients and even meals in advance.** When you return from shopping, just wash, peel, slice, and dice all your salad vegetables so you can make salads within minutes throughout the week. Store the vegetables in individual plastic bags or airtight containers in the refrigerator. Also, prepare several meals in one day. Consider making double portions and freezing half for the following week.

3. **Prepack lunch portions.** If you pack lunches, prepare single servings of thick soups or stews for lunches by spooning helpings into ziplock sandwich bags set upright in a two-cup measuring cup. Carefully press the air from the bags before closing. Mark the contents and the date before laying the bags flat in the freezer for efficient storage. Take the soup to work or school, and by lunchtime it should be thawed and ready to heat. Purchase snack-size ziplock bags to prepare servings of nuts, dried fruit, or veggies. These portions can be added to the lunch bag along with the soup and a piece of fruit for a nutritious and Daniel Fast–friendly lunch.

4. **Speed up breakfasts.** If you serve hot cereal for breakfast, prepare a divided serving dish with nuts, raisins, and other dried fruit. In the morning, serve the hot cereal in individual bowls and allow each person to garnish it as he or she desires. If you serve sliced fruit, prepare it the night before while dinner heats or after dinner along with cleanup tasks.

5. **Premake flatbreads, rice, and beans.** Your meal prep day is also a perfect time to make flatbreads or baked crackers and chips. Make each of the recipes in large batches and then store them in airtight containers to use throughout the week. Also, cook enough rice and beans to use in recipes over the next several days.

By devoting one planning and food preparation day per week, you can have nutritious and colorful meals on the table in just a few minutes, plus you will waste less food and save money by taking advantage of sales and bulk purchases. Supercharge your meal prep time by listening to teaching CDs or worship music to feed your spirit, doing laundry, and completing other household chores, so your week will run more smoothly.

With careful planning, you can prepare several meals at one time while enjoying the process. Then, as the week progresses and you experience the payoffs of your labor, you can be free of what otherwise could be a frustrating and defeating time. Give it a go. Plan your work and work your plan to enjoy a successful Daniel Fast.

Several days before you start your Daniel Fast, taper your consumption of caffeine, sugar, chemicals, and processed foods. At the same time, increase your water consumption by drinking at least a half gallon of pure water each day.

PARTICIPATE

This is where the rubber meets the road. You cross over the threshold of your Daniel Fast and move into a routine of prayer and fasting. By now you should be well prepared. You have started your fast with a high degree of expectancy and a deep commitment to honor the guidelines and the discipline.

This is a good time to journal about your fasting experience. You may also want to keep a log to track the foods you eat and the way your body is reacting to the healthier way of eating.

This book includes a twenty-one-day Daniel Fast Devotional

(see page 227) you might find useful for your study time. I also invite you to visit http://www.Daniel-Fast.com and join the mailing list so you can receive regular updates, motivational articles, more recipes, and testimonials. Check out the blog to see how others are doing on their fast and leave your own comments. We have a very sweet and supportive Daniel Fast community that spans the world. You are welcome to become part of it.

During the first few days of a fast, many people experience fatigue, headaches, leg cramps, and backaches. These are common symptoms of the detoxification process your body undergoes when you're eating foods that are good for your health. The best way to lessen these signs is to drink plenty of filtered water.

Water can also help you to manage your cravings and hunger pangs. To help me stay hydrated, I fill a pitcher with a half gallon of filtered water every day, and the first thing I do each morning is drink one full sixteen-ounce glass of water. That's 25 percent of the fluid my body needs in a normal day. I also try to drink a glass of water before each meal. Not only does this keep me hydrated, but the water also helps fill me up so I don't eat as much at meals. I try to make sure I have emptied the water pitcher by the end of the day. Since I work from my home, this is pretty easy to manage during a typical day. You may find a different system that works for you. For example, drink one sixteen-ounce glass of water in the morning, two more while on the job, and at least one more at home in the evening.

You can dress up your water by adding fresh mint or slices of lemon or cucumber to your glass. I especially like lemon because it's so refreshing in my mouth. Just make sure the water is still water rather than crossing over the line of demarcation to tea or lemonade to be consistent with the fast.

Learn to trust the Holy Spirit

When making decisions about which foods are okay and which should be avoided during the Daniel Fast, you will sometimes find yourself walking a fine line. For example, is it okay to use red wine vinegar in a salad dressing recipe when wine is not allowed on the Daniel Fast? Or if the only beverage is water, is it okay to serve fruit smoothies for breakfast? Is it okay to eat apples when they weren't even discovered until long after Daniel's time? (By the way, you can find the answers to these particular questions in the FAQs section starting on page 273.)

I've been asked these and hundreds of other questions since starting *The Daniel Fast* blog in 2007. The Daniel Fast is based on only a few Scripture references. So when you have questions where the guidelines are not definitive, seek the Holy Spirit's opinion. Listen for His still, small voice with your spiritual ears and He will guide you and direct you. Whenever I go to Him with my own questions, I have always found Him faithful to help me make decisions.

For example, several years ago I was fasting and the only soy milk I was able to find included a small amount of organic cane juice, which is a form of sugar from sugarcane. I was only going to use a little of the soy milk in a recipe, yet I found myself stumbling over the fact that it included the cane juice as an ingredient. Reason might have told me, "Oh, it's just a little bit of sugar, and besides, you already have the soy milk and it would be a shame to throw it away."

But when I stood in my kitchen and asked the Holy Spirit for His opinion, I felt certain His still, small voice was telling me to forgo the soy milk and find an alternative. He seemed to be saying that being strict in this circumstance would help hone my discernment and decision-making skills. So I didn't use the soy milk and instead gave it to a friend. Now I am able to find unsweetened soy milk and use it in my recipes.

Your fast is yours, others' fasts are theirs

I receive many e-mails from frustrated spouses, usually wives, who are angry with their partners who aren't doing the fast the way they think they should. The spouse won't adhere to the fasting guidelines or wants to change them to meet his or her likes. Some couples have written wanting me to settle their argument about what is okay to eat and what isn't. This is not a hat I'm willing to wear, so though I try to provide answers to specific questions about the fast, I mostly try to encourage people to be supportive and loving toward their spouses, and also to understand that we are each responsible for our own fast. It's best to focus on our fast rather than on someone else's.

I know this can be tough, but this experience offers another life lesson. How do we react when we see people behaving in ways that we consider wrong? Are we quick to point out their mistake? Do we get mad when they don't do things the way we think they should be done? Do we call our friends and tell them all about it?

We can be supportive and helpful and in a caring, gentle way show people a mistake they might be unknowingly making *if* we are guided by the Spirit to do so. But unless I am very sure God wants me to be His messenger, I've found that the best action we can take is to pray and then support the areas where people are successful and let them deal with the areas where they might be weak.

If you encounter this matter, use it as a learning experience for your relationship and your own skills. Seek the guidance of the Holy Spirit and study the Word of God to see what it has to say. And stay focused on your fast, being a positive witness as you grow in the ways of Christ through the discipline of prayer and fasting.

Know when to take a break

Will there be times when you must forgo the fast or temporarily pause from it? Yes—for example, when unexpected circumstances such as an emergency or serious health issue strikes. Suddenly, staying on the fast pales in comparison to the crisis.

Last year I received an e-mail from a mother whose daughter had just been killed in a tragic car accident. Clearly, this was a time when the fast should be stopped so family members could attend to the pressing needs of the situation.

Sometimes we need to take a break for other reasons as well. I recall a time when I took a twenty-four-hour "time-out" from my Daniel Fast. I live about a hundred miles from my son, Dawit, and his wife. I adopted Dawit from Ethiopia when he was just seven years old. When he was a young adult, he went back to Ethiopia for a year, and while there, he married a lovely woman. They settled in Seattle, in the midst of the Ethiopian community. One day I drove over to Seattle to visit them. I was fasting at the time, but I wasn't too concerned. Many Ethiopian dishes are appropriate for the Daniel Fast. Plus, I knew I could always eat salads and rice and drink water, so I didn't think it was necessary to make any special arrangements. I was excited to get there, because I hadn't seen my son and his wife for a while.

Let me set the stage a little more. In the Ethiopian community, parents and elders are highly honored; children and young people always defer to their parents and anyone senior in age. I was raised with similar values, but for Ethiopians honoring parents is deeply ingrained in their culture, their way of life, and their thinking.

I arrived at my son and daughter-in-law's apartment late in the day, and as soon as I entered I could smell the scrumptious aroma of Ethiopian food. My daughter-in-law, Rodas, is an excellent cook, and I especially like the Ethiopian cuisine. The sauces are tomato-based with a lot of spices, so they are Daniel Fast–friendly. I could also eat the unleavened Ethiopian bread called *injera*, which is not only a kind of flatbread, it's also an eating utensil. In Ethiopia, this spongy, sour flatbread is used to scoop up meat, chicken, and vegetable stews. Injera usually lines the common plate on which the stews are served, soaking up their juices as the meal progresses. When this edible container is eaten, the meal is officially over.

When dinnertime arrived, we all gathered at the dining table. Rodas brought the injera, a split pea stew, cooked greens, and one other dish.

"Here, Mom. I made this especially for you," she said, presenting me with a steaming hot dish filled with lamb in a savory Ethiopian sauce.

I had to make a quick decision: should I turn the food down or accept the kindness my daughter-in-law is giving to me? I lodged an instant prayer to the Holy Spirit, perceived His direction, accepted the act of kindness, and ate the meal. Love trumped my fast, and I sensed a peace about the situation.

Later that evening, Rodas presented me with a traditional Ethiopian coffee ceremony, also an act of respect and friendship toward the recipient. Coffee was discovered in Ethiopia in the ninth century, and the beverage plays a central part in this deeply rooted tradition. A coffee ceremony is a pretty big deal, and I felt honored that Rodas wanted to bestow this service to me. The coffee servings are small, but strong and sweet. I accepted one cup (usually three are consumed), and again felt peace about the decision. The next morning I enjoyed fresh fruit for breakfast, and then I returned home, where I resumed the Daniel Fast for the remainder of the days.

When you fast, you may find yourself facing similar dilemmas. I believe a key is to check your heart and make sure the reason you push the "pause button" is coming from your spirit and you are not just giving in to a craving for a self-motivated reason. In most cases I can avoid these situations. And over all my years of fasting, it's the rare occasion when I have paused my fast. But I wanted to include this example so you don't beat yourself up if you defer due to love, respect, or some other act of kindness or when unexpected situations arise.

With that said, there are also many times when friends ask me to a meal at their home and I tell them I am on the Daniel Fast. I explain that there is no need for special arrangements or to change what will be eaten. I go on to clarify that I am totally satisfied with a vegetable salad and drinking water, and if that works, I will be happy to attend.

End the Daniel Fast carefully

If you have been fasting for an extended period of time, you will want to be careful when it ends and you begin to reintroduce foods into your diet. Keep in mind that you have been giving your body foods that are good for it and that cause your digestive tract to operate at optimal levels. You also have not had processed foods, proteins that are harder to digest, caffeine, or sugar.

It's tempting to end your fast by feasting on foods you've been denied for so long. But the result will most likely be a massive rebuttal from your body in the form of cramping, bloating, gas, and stomach upset. Your body will be much happier if you slowly reintroduce foods and beverages to your diet.

PRAISE GOD AND PROCESS

When you complete your Daniel Fast, you will want to review your experience. What did you learn? Are there habits that you want to carry forward into your everyday life?

I receive many words of testimony from men and women all over the world about the amazing benefits of their fasts. There are two praises that are most often mentioned. First, men and women discover a deeper and more intimate relationship with God when they develop daily habits of meeting with their Father and studying His Word. They receive many answers as they discover the power of bringing everything to the Lord in prayer. And I rejoice with them as they celebrate the deep and abiding relationship they now have with their Creator.

Second, the health benefits of the Daniel Fast are significant for many, particularly those who suffer from debilitating diseases or obesity! Words cannot express the delight I experience when I read messages from men and women who say they have never been able to diet before, but the Daniel Fast has shown them a new and healthy way of life. Many are able to stop some or all of the medications they've been taking as their bodies respond to nutritious food and a balanced, healthy diet. They also report that their doctors are delighted when they see the difference. (Remember to always stay under the guidance of your health-care provider if you have a medical issue.)

By the end of your fast, you will have proven to yourself that you can change your eating habits. Why not consider making healthy long-term changes to your day-to-day eating plan? Eat vegan meals several times a week. Think about switching to alternative natural sweeteners such as honey, Stevia, or agave nectar and eating only whole grains rather than processed foods. Continue to keep your body well hydrated by drinking at least a half gallon of water each day, and exercise portion control.

Take a few minutes and do a "before and after" comparison. If you really struggled during the fast, open a conversation with yourself and try to get to the bottom of the reasons things didn't turn out the way you had hoped.

Whether you felt the fast was successful or not, what will you do the next time you fast to make your experience even better? These are all important questions to ask yourself. You may want to jot down some notes and put them in a file or store them in the pages of this book for next time around.

Take some time to thank your Father for the experience and the lessons He has taught you. Consider writing down at least ten praises, and then bless the Lord by thanking Him for them.

The Bible says, "But we all, with unveiled face, beholding as in a mirror the glory of the Lord, are being transformed into the same image from glory to glory, just as by the Spirit of the Lord" (2 Corinthians 3:18).

During your fast you have learned empowering lessons about living by faith and walking in the Spirit. As you move into your normal way of life, bring with it the lessons you've learned. Create a "new normal" with your increased spiritual awareness, your new habits of consistently spending time in prayer and study, and the healthy dietary choices you've learned.

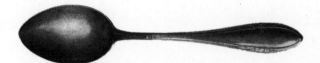

PART TWO

Step into a new way of life as you
offer yourself unto the
Lord as a spiritual offering.

The Daniel Fast Food List

AFTER ANSWERING HUNDREDS of questions about the Daniel Fast on the blog, I created the following food guidelines. I use the statement "including but not limited to" as a way to communicate that many similar but unlisted foods may also be included. Even though "Asian pears," for example, are not listed under fruits, they are allowed because they are fruit.

Also, folks on the blog laughed at me when I started "shouting" in all capitals to readers, "READ THE LABEL" after answering hundreds and hundreds of questions about purchasing packaged, canned, or bottled foods. When you consider a food item, take a look at the ingredient list included on the label. It's usually near or under the nutritional information. The acceptable foods must be *sweetener-free*, *chemical-free*, and *consistent* with the food lists below.

FOODS TO INCLUDE IN YOUR DIET
DURING THE DANIEL FAST

All fruits. These can be fresh, frozen, dried, juiced, or canned. Fruits include but are not limited to apples, apricots, bananas, blackberries, blueberries, boysenberries, cantaloupe, cherries, cranberries, dates, figs, grapefruit, grapes, guava, honeydew melon, kiwi, lemons, limes, mangoes, nectarines, oranges, papayas, peaches, pears, pineapples, plums, prunes, raisins, raspberries, strawberries, tangelos, tangerines, and watermelon.

All vegetables. These can be fresh, frozen, dried, juiced, or canned. Vegetables include but are not limited to artichokes, asparagus, avocados, beets, bok choy, broccoli, brussels sprouts, cabbage, carrots, cauliflower, celery, chili peppers, collard greens, corn, cucumbers, eggplant, garlic, gingerroot, green beans, jicama, kale, leeks, lettuce, mushrooms, mustard greens, okra, olives, onions, parsley, parsnips, peppers, potatoes, radishes, rutabagas, scallions, shallots, spinach, sprouts, squashes, sweet potatoes, tomatoes, tomato paste, turnips, water chestnuts, watercress, yams, and zucchini. Veggie burgers are an option if you are not allergic to soy.

All whole grains. These include but are not limited to barley, brown rice, corn flour, cornmeal, grits, millet, oat bran, oats, popcorn, quinoa, rice cakes, wheat germ, whole wheat, whole wheat pasta, and whole wheat tortillas.

All nuts and seeds. These include but are not limited to almonds, cashews, coconut, flax seeds, pecans, peanuts, pine nuts, poppy seeds, sesame seeds, and walnuts. Nut butters such as peanut butter and tahini (sesame seed paste) may be included.

All legumes. These can be canned or dried. Legumes include but are not limited to black beans, black-eyed peas, cannellini beans, chickpeas, dried beans, kidney beans, lentils, lima beans, navy beans, pinto beans, split peas, and white beans.

All quality oils. These include but are not limited to canola, coconut, grape seed, olive, peanut, and sesame.

Water. Distilled water, filtered water, spring water, or other pure waters.

Soy foods. These include tofu (all kinds), TVP (textured vegetable protein), and other soy products.

Condiments and cooking ingredients. Adobo sauce, cilantro, herbs, mustard (unsweetened), salt, seasonings, soynnaise, spices, TVP, vanilla, and vegetable broth. You can use small amounts of fruit juices as ingredients in dishes (apple juice, lemon juice, lime juice, orange juice, pineapple juice).

FOODS TO RESTRICT ON THE DANIEL FAST

Exclude **all meat and animal products** such as beef, lamb, pork, poultry, and fish.

Exclude **all dairy products** such as milk, cheese, cream, butter, and eggs.

Exclude **all sweeteners** such as sugar, raw sugar, honey, syrups, molasses, and cane juice.

Exclude **all leavened bread** such as Ezekiel Bread (most of which contains yeast and honey), pretzels, pita bread, and other baked goods made with leavening agents.

Exclude **all refined and processed food products** that contain such ingredients as artificial flavorings, food additives, chemicals, white rice, white flour, or artificial preservatives.

Exclude **all deep-fried foods** such as potato chips, French fries, and corn chips.

Exclude **all solid fats** such as shortening, margarine, lard, and foods high in fat.

Exclude **all nonwater beverages** such as coffee, tea, herbal teas, carbonated beverages, energy drinks, and alcohol.

Remember, READ THE LABELS to know all the ingredients included in prepared foods!

STOCKING YOUR PANTRY

An important key to success for the Daniel Fast is having easy access to the foods you need to stay within the guidelines. Here are some items to keep on hand:

- Fresh fruit: Apples, bananas, blueberries, grapefruit, lemons, limes, oranges.
- Fresh vegetables: Bell peppers (green and red), cucumber, green lettuce, scallions (aka green onions), yellow onions,

tomatoes (I know tomatoes are really a fruit, but it seems we usually use them as a vegetable).

- Canned foods: Beans in various varieties (black, kidney, pinto, and chickpeas), jalapeño peppers, pineapple juice, tomato sauce, diced tomatoes.

- Frozen foods: Corn, peas, mixed vegetables, stir-fry vegetables, apple juice concentrate.

- Whole grains and legumes: Brown rice, oatmeal, muesli, green peas, lentils.

- Dried fruit: Raisins, apricots, dates.

- Miscellaneous: Peanut butter, rice cakes, walnuts, almonds, soy milk.

Eat foods that work for you! Some fruits, vegetables, healthy fats, and grains are very good at speeding up your metabolism. Some of the best vegetables are asparagus, beets, broccoli, cabbage, carrots, spinach, and tomatoes. Among the best fruits are apples, blueberries, citrus fruits, melons, and pears. Nuts and nut butters are good in moderation, and brown rice, barley, and oats are among the whole grains that rev up your metabolism.

In the next section, you'll find a number of recipes that incorporate these ingredients. In addition to the items above, I keep several items in my pantry for when I want a fast and easy breakfast:

Ezekiel 4:9 Sprouted Whole Grain Cereal. This is a boxed breakfast cereal that you can purchase in the natural foods section of most supermarkets or at health food stores. The thing that makes this cereal so perfect for the Daniel Fast is that it doesn't have any added sweeteners, only whole grains with a little salt. It's more expensive than typical boxed cereals (each serving costs about seventy cents), but the ingredients are so much better for you and of greater value for your body. A half-cup serving of this whole grain cereal contains 0 grams of sugar and 8 grams of protein or 17 percent of the daily requirement. Compare this with

Trix, a boxed cereal made by General Mills, with 13 grams of sugar and only 1 gram of protein per serving. I eat Ezekiel 4:9 cereal almost every day, whether I am fasting or not. I just add a handful of fresh blueberries, sometimes a sliced banana, and then top it with one-half cup unsweetened soy milk. So good!

Bob's Red Mill Old Country Style Muesli. Bob's Red Mill products are also found in the natural foods section of most supermarkets or at health food stores. The muesli is just like the kind developed in the late 1800s by a Swiss nutritionist and is a blend of whole grains, dried fruit, nuts, and seeds. Serve it hot or cold (I like it hot) along with a sliced banana and soy milk for a great start to your day.

Zoom. This takes me back to my childhood. My father was a school principal by profession and the chief breakfast chef at home. Many mornings he would cook a pot of Zoom, which is 100 percent whole wheat. That's it! Read the ingredient list on the box and you see "Whole Wheat." It cooks quickly and is delicious and nutritious with some fresh or dried fruit and a little unsweetened soy milk.

These cereal products, along with unsweetened soy milk (substitute rice or almond milk if you prefer), dried fruit, nuts, and fresh fruit make for a delicious breakfast. You'll be eating more in line with how our Creator planned it—whole foods packed with vitamins and minerals to nourish your body.

By the way, don't be surprised when you lose your sweet tooth on the Daniel Fast. My mouth used to pucker when I ate cereal with only fresh blueberries and a little unsweetened soy milk so I would add a banana to balance the flavors. But now I taste the sweetness in the blueberries and am delighted with the simple meal.

TOO MUCH OF A GOOD THING CAN STILL BE BAD FOR YOU!

Just because you will be eating foods that are good for your body doesn't mean that you should eat in excess. Portion control is important whenever we eat, and especially during the Daniel Fast.

I'm often asked, "How much should I eat on the Daniel Fast?" I respond by explaining that even though we can eat some foods, we are fasting. So three modest meals and two snacks each day is reasonable.

This is also a good time to check in with the Holy Spirit. Ask Him if you are eating too much, if you are giving in to your cravings for more instead of using self-control, which is a powerful fruit of the Spirit.

Look at the Nutritional Facts label to learn how much a serving represents. For example, a serving of cooked oatmeal is one-half cup; a serving of fresh fruit is a medium-sized apple or one banana; and a serving of beans is three heaped tablespoons full. Finally, consider calories. For most healthy people, a healthy caloric intake per day is between 2,200 and 2,800 calories, depending on gender and size.[11]

Daniel Fast Recipes

Breakfasts

When many people think of breakfast, they envision pancakes, waffles, bacon and eggs, or sugary cereals. However, these foods are all restricted on the Daniel Fast. The good news is that on the next few pages there are many very nutritious and pleasant breakfasts you can make for your family. Don't be surprised if you change your morning eating habits once you've enjoyed these healthy meals.

Dried Fruit and Almond Granola

Granola is a perfect breakfast choice on the Daniel Fast. But most granola found in supermarkets includes sweeteners or other ingredients not included on the Daniel Fast. So making a big batch of this easy (and very affordable) recipe is a smart move. Plus it's so nutritious and filling.

INGREDIENTS

- 2 cups rolled oats
- ½ cup shredded coconut
- ½ cup sliced almonds
- 3 tablespoons vegetable oil (such as canola oil)
- ½ cup chopped dried fruit (apples, figs, apricots, etc.)
- ½ cup raisins

1. Preheat oven to 350 degrees.
2. Combine oats, coconut, and almonds in a large baking dish. Drizzle with oil and toss until well blended. Bake in preheated oven for 15–20 minutes, tossing every 5 minutes, until lightly toasted.
3. Allow mixture to cool slightly before mixing in dried fruit and raisins.
4. Store in airtight container and serve with soy milk, fresh fruit, and/or fruit juice.

Makes 4 cups (about 8 servings)

Apple Pie Oatmeal

This recipe is a tasty way to prepare and serve a great meal for yourself and your family. Rolled oats are an excellent food choice for breakfast because they provide valuable protein, stave off hunger for a long period of time, and provide beneficial fiber to do good work in your body!

INGREDIENTS

- 4 cups water
- ¼ teaspoon salt
- 2 cups rolled oats
- ½ teaspoon Apple Pie Spice (see recipe below)
- ¼ cup chopped apple

1. Bring water to a boil in medium saucepan over medium-high heat. Add salt and when dissolved, stir in oats and Apple Pie Spice. Reduce heat and continue to cook for 4 minutes.
2. Add chopped apple and cook for 1–2 more minutes until oats are cooked.
3. Serve in individual bowls with unsweetened soy milk, if desired.

Makes 4 servings

Apple Pie Spice

- ½ teaspoon ground cinnamon
- ¼ teaspoon ground nutmeg
- ⅛ teaspoon ground allspice
- ⅛ teaspoon ground cardamom

Combine all ingredients. If making a larger batch, store in an airtight container.
Use with Apple Pie Oatmeal or other recipes that call for Apple Pie Spice.

Banana Wheat Bran Cereal

When I was growing up, my father was often the one who prepared school-morning breakfasts. The most common fare was hot oatmeal and Zoom, a whole wheat cereal made by Krusteaz, a division of Continental Mills. Little did I know that good ole Dad was serving such healthy meals. Wheat bran is packed with fiber and healthy nutrients. Plus the cereal is perfect for Daniel Fast breakfasts. This recipe adds bananas, but you can be creative and add other fruits to suit your taste.

INGREDIENTS

- 2⅔ cups water
- ½ teaspoon salt
- 1⅓ cups Zoom Whole Wheat Cereal
- 1 cup mashed ripe banana
- 1 teaspoon cinnamon
- ¼ cup slivered almonds

1. Bring water to a boil in a covered saucepan; add salt.

2. Stir in Zoom and reduce heat; continue to boil for 1 minute, stirring frequently.

3. Cover and remove from heat. Let stand 1 minute before serving.

4. Stir in banana, cinnamon, and almonds and serve with unsweetened soy, rice, or almond milk, if desired.

Makes 4 servings

Four Grain Muesli

Muesli is a breakfast cereal of Swiss origin, made of uncooked grains, nuts, and dried fruits. It may be eaten with hot or cold soy milk, fruit juice, or applesauce. This muesli recipe uses four grains as well as some dried fruit and nuts and seeds. Making your own muesli saves money and is so easy!

INGREDIENTS

- 4½ cups rolled oats
- ½ cup wheat germ
- ½ cup wheat bran
- ½ cup oat bran
- 1 cup raisins

- ¼ cup finely chopped dates
- ½ cup chopped walnuts
- ¼ cup raw sunflower seeds

1. In a large mixing bowl, combine oats, wheat germ, wheat bran, oat bran, dried fruit, nuts, and seeds. Mix well.

2. Store muesli in an airtight container and it will keep nicely for 2 months in your cupboard.

3. Serve muesli either hot or cold with fresh fruit and soy milk.

Hot Muesli Instructions: Add ½ cup muesli to ½ cup water or soy milk; bring to a boil. Simmer for 3–5 minutes. You can also microwave muesli in a large bowl on high for 3–5 minutes, stirring once halfway through.

Cold Muesli Instructions: Soak ½ cup muesli in ½ cup soy milk or fruit juice for 5–10 minutes, or soak overnight in the refrigerator.

Makes 2 servings

Quick and Easy Muesli

This is the "fast food" version of muesli. Be creative by adding the whole grain cereals you have on hand or especially like. The same goes for your choice of dried fruit and nuts or seeds. See what you have in your cupboard, blend the ingredients, and you have a simple breakfast cereal.

INGREDIENTS

- 2 cups rolled oats (or any combination of whole grains you prefer)
- ½ cup chopped dried fruit (apples, dates, figs, apricots, etc.)
- ½ cup raisins
- ½ cup nuts or seeds

1. Combine all ingredients in a large bowl (if desired, grind in a food processor until the ingredients are of a uniform texture).

2. Store muesli in an airtight container and it will keep nicely for 2 months in your cupboard.

3. Serve muesli either hot or cold with fresh fruit and soy milk.

Makes 3 cups (about 6 servings)

Yummy Brown Rice with Apple

Renee Hastings, member of our Daniel Fast community, sent this breakfast idea to me, and the recipe has become one of my favorites. The brown rice is a great way to start the day with added fiber. The chopped apple and coconut oil provide a sweetness and rich flavor making the dish delicious.

INGREDIENTS

- 2 tablespoons coconut oil
- 4 cups cooked brown rice
- 2 cups chopped apple (choose a sweet variety)
- Cinnamon (optional)

1. Heat oil in a saucepan or skillet over medium-high heat; add cooked rice and chopped apple and stir to blend well. Reduce heat to medium-low.

2. Continue to heat, stirring often until all ingredients are hot. If desired, add cinnamon and stir well. Serve with or without unsweetened soy milk.

Makes 4 servings

Basic Tofu Scramble

If you have never eaten tofu, this is an excellent way to introduce the protein soy product to your diet. One of the unique qualities of tofu is that it soaks up the flavors of the foods that it's with, so sautéing tofu with onions and bell peppers allows the flavor to expand. The texture of tofu is similar to egg whites in this recipe, so it's a winner on that front as well!

INGREDIENTS

- 2 tablespoons olive oil
- 1 yellow onion, diced
- 1 green bell pepper, diced
- 1 block tofu, drained, pressed, and cut into 1-inch cubes
- 1 teaspoon garlic powder
- 1 teaspoon onion powder
- 1 tablespoon soy sauce
- ½ teaspoon turmeric (optional)
- 1 tablespoon chopped fresh parsley

1. Heat oil in a large skillet over medium-high heat. Add onion, pepper, and tofu and sauté for 3–5 minutes, stirring often.

2. Stir in garlic powder, onion powder, soy sauce, and turmeric; reduce heat to medium and cook 5–7 more minutes, stirring frequently (add more oil if needed).

3. Add fresh parsley just before serving.

4. Serve tofu scramble with fresh fruit or wrap in a warmed flour tortilla with a bit of salsa for a breakfast burrito.

Makes 4 servings

Curried Tofu Scramble

Packed with flavor, protein, and vitamins, this quick recipe is a perfect option for the Daniel Fast. Serve with fresh fruit for a delightful meal.

INGREDIENTS

- 1 teaspoon olive oil
- 1 onion, diced
- 3 cloves garlic, minced
- 1 block firm or extra firm tofu, drained, pressed, and crumbled
- 1 teaspoon curry powder
- ½ teaspoon turmeric
- ½ teaspoon cumin (optional)
- Salt and pepper to taste
- 2 tomatoes, diced
- 1 bunch fresh spinach

1. Heat the oil in a large skillet over medium high heat; add onion and garlic; sauté for 3–5 minutes or until onion is soft.

2. Add tofu, curry powder, turmeric, cumin, salt, pepper, and tomatoes; cook, stirring often, for another 5 minutes until tofu is hot and cooked; add more oil if needed.

3. Add spinach and cook 1–2 minutes, just until wilted.

4. Serve hot.

Makes 4 servings

Tomato and Green Pepper Tofu Scramble

This is a great recipe to introduce tofu to your diet, especially if you like tomatoes. A bland form of protein becomes rich in flavor!

INGREDIENTS

- 2 tablespoons olive oil
- 1 yellow onion, diced
- 1 green bell pepper, cored and sliced into bite-size pieces
- 2 garlic cloves, minced
- 1 block firm tofu, cut into 1-inch cubes
- 1 cup tomato juice or sauce
- 1 tomato, seeded and diced
- 1 teaspoon garlic powder
- 1 teaspoon onion powder
- ½ teaspoon liquid smoke
- 1 tablespoon soy sauce
- ½ teaspoon turmeric
- ¼ teaspoon ground cumin
- Salt and pepper to taste

1. Heat olive oil in a large skillet over medium heat; sauté onion, bell pepper, and garlic for 3 minutes or until onion is soft.

2. Add the tofu and the tomato juice. Simmer until the peppers are cooked.

3. Stir in tomato, garlic powder, onion powder, liquid smoke, soy sauce, turmeric, and cumin; cook until all ingredients are well heated; add more oil if necessary.

4. Adjust seasoning with salt and pepper. Serve hot along with side of fresh fruit or wrap in chapati and garnish with salsa for a breakfast burrito.

Makes 4 servings

Tofu-Veggie Breakfast Scramble

This recipe is a great choice for those busy mornings when you want a protein-rich hot breakfast that is also colorful and full of flavor. Be creative with this recipe, customizing it to your own preferences.

INGREDIENTS

- 1 tablespoon olive oil
- 1 block firm tofu, patted dry and mashed

- 1 cup of your favorite fresh or frozen vegetables, such as broccoli, sweet peppers, onions, mushrooms, or tomatoes
- ⅛ teaspoon turmeric
- 1 teaspoon onion powder
- ½ teaspoon salt

1. Heat the oil in a sauté pan over medium heat. Add the tofu and heat for about 3 minutes.

2. Add the vegetables, turmeric, onion powder, and salt; stir and cook for about 5 minutes or until vegetables are just tender.

3. Adjust seasoning and serve.

Makes 4 servings

Potato and Scallion Breakfast Frittata

This recipe takes some time, but it's a great breakfast meal for weekends on the Daniel Fast. I like to change the potatoes, depending on my schedule and what I have available. For fast meals, frozen shredded potatoes are great. But my favorite way to prepare this meal is to use chopped new potatoes.

INGREDIENTS

- ¼ cup olive oil
- 1 onion, finely chopped
- 4–5 scallions, chopped, with the green and white parts separated
- 4 cloves garlic, minced
- 2 medium potatoes, shredded (or 2 cups of frozen shredded potatoes)
- 2 teaspoons salt, divided
- ½ teaspoon freshly ground black pepper, divided
- 2 blocks firm tofu, cut into chunks
- 2–3 tablespoons soy sauce

1. Preheat the oven to 350 degrees.

2. Heat the olive oil in a large skillet over medium heat. Add the onion and the white part of the scallions; sauté for 2–3 minutes; add the garlic and heat for another 30 seconds.

3. Increase the heat to medium-high and add the potatoes, 1 teaspoon of the salt, and ¼ teaspoon of the pepper; cook for 10–15 minutes, tossing the potatoes regularly until they are well browned.

4. Place the tofu, soy sauce, and the remaining salt and pepper in a food processor; blend until creamy.

5. Pour creamy mixture and the green part of the scallions over the fried potatoes and mix. Pour this mixture into a large, oiled pie or tart pan.

6. Bake for 30–40 minutes or until the center is firm. Invert the frittata onto a warmed serving plate.

Makes 4 servings

Drew's Breakfast Burritos

Drew and Erin Bishop are friends of mine. I meet with Erin almost every week over coffee for "Christian girl talk." She's a full-time vegan, but her husband Drew and their two children eat a more typical diet. Drew shared this recipe that he found helpful the last time he was on the Daniel Fast. There is lots of protein in these healthy bundles!

INGREDIENTS

- 1–2 tablespoons olive oil
- ½ cup finely diced yellow or white onion
- 2 cloves garlic, finely minced
- 2 cups cooked brown rice
- 1 cup extra firm tofu, crumbled
- 3 Roma tomatoes, seeded and diced
- ½ cup chopped fresh cilantro
- 2–5 serrano chiles, seeded and finely chopped (optional)
- 2 teaspoons fresh lime juice
- 1 teaspoon salt
- 4 whole wheat burritos

1. Heat olive oil in a skillet over medium heat; add the onion and garlic; sauté until soft, about 3 minutes. Add the brown rice and tofu and stir until well heated.

2. Stir in the tomatoes, cilantro, and chiles, mixing until all the ingredients are well heated.

3. Just before serving, stir in the lime juice and salt; spoon in equal portions onto whole wheat burritos.

Makes 4 servings

Home Fried Breakfast Potatoes

These spicy home fried potatoes round out a hearty breakfast meal. Pair with a tofu scramble, sliced fresh fruit, or black bean salsa.

INGREDIENTS

- Salted water (for boiling potatoes)
- 4 red potatoes
- 3 tablespoons olive oil, divided
- 1 yellow onion, chopped
- 1 green bell pepper, seeded and chopped
- 1 teaspoon salt
- ¾ teaspoon paprika
- ¼ teaspoon freshly ground black pepper
- ¼ cup chopped fresh Italian parsley

1. Bring a large pot of salted water to a boil over high heat. Add potatoes and cook until just tender, about 15 minutes (be careful not to overcook). Drain, cool, and cut into ½-inch cubes.

2. Heat 1 tablespoon olive oil in a large skillet over medium-high heat. Add onion and green pepper; cook until soft, stirring often, about 5 minutes. Transfer to a plate, and set aside.

3. Heat remaining 2 tablespoons of oil in the same skillet over medium-high heat. Add potato cubes, salt, paprika, and black pepper. Cook until potatoes are browned, stirring often, about 10 minutes.

4. Add onions, green peppers, and parsley; cook for another minute or until all ingredients are well heated.

5. Adjust seasoning and serve hot.

Makes 4 servings

Fruit and Vegetable Smoothies

Smoothies are a popular quick meal and a useful way to consume valuable nutrients. Several recipes are provided here, but be creative as you plan your smoothie. Use local organic fruits and vegetables whenever possible. Also, when local produce is not available, consider frozen options, as they often retain more of the food value than fresh varieties that are picked before they ripen and then are stored for long periods of time before they reach the grocery stores. Here are some tips and tricks to a great smoothie.

1. The key to a perfect smoothie is the correct proportions of fresh fruit, frozen fruit, and juice. (See recipes for proportions.)

2. To balance flavors, use a mix of tart fruits and sweet fruits.

3. The more frozen fruits you use, the thicker the smoothie will be. You can thin the mixture with ice cubes, soy milk, or fruit juice.

4. If you don't want the smoothie watered down, choose juice or soy milk to thin the consistency.

5. Fresh fruit and juice mix easier, resulting in a smoother consistency.

6. Ground flaxseed is a great fiber source and does not alter the taste of the smoothie.

7. Invest in a good blender if you plan to make smoothies often.

8. If you plan to add protein powders to your smoothie, be sure to check the ingredients to make sure there are no dairy, sweeteners, or chemicals. Add the protein powder at the end of the blending process or the smoothie may become too frothy.

9. After blending, add coarsely chopped frozen grapes as "sweet ice cubes."

10. Serve your smoothie with a small handful of raw nuts for a quick and nutritious breakfast.

A healthy breakfast is the most important meal of the day and is important to start the day off right. Get creative and become a smoothie expert!

Following are some tasty combinations to get you started:
Tropical: Fresh banana and frozen mango with pineapple juice
Very Berry: Fresh or frozen blueberries, raspberries, and strawberries with pomegranate juice
Peachy Dreams: Fresh or frozen strawberries and peaches with orange juice

Then experiment with other combinations or ingredients:
Try using frozen blueberries, mixed berries, peaches, or raspberries in place of the frozen strawberries.
Pineapple, pomegranate, or grape juice are flavorful alternatives to orange juice.
Consider ripe peaches, mangoes, or pineapple in place of the banana.

Why Are Smoothies Allowed?
The only acceptable beverage on the Daniel Fast is water (see Daniel 1). However, smoothies are allowed since they are considered a "liquid meal" rather than a beverage.

Single Serving Fruit Smoothie

This basic fruit smoothie recipe is a great option for breakfast with your favorite seasonal fruits.

INGREDIENTS

- 1 cup unsweetened soy milk or silken tofu
- 1 ripe banana, broken into chunks
- ½ cup of your favorite fresh or frozen fruit (strawberries, peaches, pitted cherries)
- Pinch of cinnamon
- 2–3 ice cubes

1. Place all ingredients (except ice cubes) in a blender and puree until smooth.
2. Add ice cubes one at a time to reach desired consistency.
3. Serve cold.

Makes 1 serving

Strawberry Oatmeal Smoothie

Adding soy milk and oatmeal to a breakfast smoothie is an inventive way to add even more protein and fiber to your meal, which is so important in a healthy diet.

INGREDIENTS

- 1 cup unsweetened soy milk
- ½ cup rolled oats
- 1 banana, broken into chunks
- 14 fresh or frozen strawberries
- ½ teaspoon pure vanilla extract
- 2 tablespoons apple or pineapple juice

1. In a blender, combine soy milk, oats, banana, and strawberries.
2. Add vanilla and enough juice for desired consistency; blend until smooth.
3. Pour into glasses and serve cold.

Makes 2 servings

Berry Banana Smoothie

This smoothie is light, but still very filling. For additional nutrients, consider adding fresh or frozen spinach. The great news is that you won't taste the spinach, and the deep color of the blueberries masks the green color.

INGREDIENTS

- 1 ripe banana, broken into chunks
- 1 cup frozen blueberries
- 1 cup unsweetened almond, rice, or soy milk
- 1 tablespoon ground flaxseed
- ½ teaspoon cinnamon (optional)
- ½ cup fresh or frozen spinach (optional)
- 2–3 ice cubes

1. Place the banana, blueberries, almond milk, flaxseed, cinnamon, and spinach (if desired) in a blender; blend until smooth.

2. Add ice to reach desired consistency and serve cold.

Makes 1 serving

Tropical Fruit and Tofu Smoothie

This is another option for a fruit smoothie for a family breakfast. Feel free to change the ingredients to meet your tastes.

INGREDIENTS

- 1 cup fresh or frozen fruit, such as mango, papaya, or pineapple
- 3 cups apple juice, bottled or made from concentrate
- 1 cup silken tofu
- ¼ cup lemon juice
- 12 ice cubes (or the number needed to reach desired consistency)

1. Place the fruit, apple juice, tofu, lemon juice, and a few ice cubes in a blender. Blend until smooth.

2. Add ice cubes and blend to reach desired consistency.

Makes 4 servings

East Indian Mango Lassi Smoothie

Mango lassi is a type of smoothie commonly made in India. However, the main ingredient is yogurt. This recipe is close to the classic lassi using tofu, mango, orange juice, and a little lemon juice to simulate the familar tang of yogurt. You can substitute pineapple or other tropical fruits for this healthy liquid breakfast meal.

INGREDIENTS

- 1 cup fresh or frozen mango chunks
- 3 cups unsweetened orange juice
- 1 cup silken tofu
- 3 tablespoons lemon juice
- 12 ice cubes (or the number needed to reach desired consistency)

1. Place the mango, orange juice, tofu, lemon juice, and 6 ice cubes in a blender; puree until smooth and frothy.

2. Add more ice cubes to create the desired consistency. Serve immediately.

Makes 4 servings

Main Dishes

Lunches and dinners will require planning and preparation time. But you can streamline your efforts by cooking double portions and freezing them for a later meal or setting aside a "cooking day" to prepare and store several meals at one time.

You will save countless hours by planning your meals at least one week in advance and then using your time in the kitchen wisely by preparing meals ahead and multitasking. Your kitchen time is also a perfect opportunity to listen to teachings from your favorite Bible teachers or pastors. I have a small CD player in my kitchen that I use when I am preparing meals or cleaning. Not only does the time pass quickly, but I am learning and feeding my spirit at the same time. I also listen to the same teaching series several times to get truth deeply rooted in my spirit.

Black Bean, Corn, and Brown Rice Stuffed Peppers

We are so accustomed to eating meat, poultry, or chicken as a main course that it can be challenging on the Daniel Fast to prepare something that seems as substantial. This recipe definitely fits the bill! I love these little gems, and the beans and rice form a complete protein so it's satisfying all around! This is also one of those recipes that's even better the next day as the flavors fuse in all the ingredients.

INGREDIENTS

- 2 cans (15 ounces each) black beans, drained
- 3 cups cooked brown rice, divided
- 1 cup frozen corn kernels, thawed
- 2 scallions, sliced
- ¼ cup chopped fresh cilantro
- 2 tablespoons extra-virgin olive oil
- 2 tablespoons fresh lime juice
- 1 clove garlic, minced
- Salt and freshly ground pepper to taste
- 2–3 large bell peppers, cut in half lengthwise and cored
- 2 cups 100% vegetable or tomato juice

1. Preheat the oven to 350 degrees.

2. Using a large bowl, gently combine the beans, 1 cup of the brown rice, corn, scallions, cilantro, olive oil, lime juice, and garlic. Season with salt and pepper to taste.

3. Place the pepper halves in a large glass baking dish and stuff them with the bean and rice mixture.

4. Carefully spoon some of the juice over each stuffed pepper, trying not to disrupt the filling. Pour the remainder of the juice into the dish. Cover with foil and bake for 45–60 minutes.

5. To serve, place about ½ cup of brown rice on each plate, spoon some of the juice from the baking dish on the rice, and then place a stuffed pepper on top of the rice.

6. Serve hot.

Makes 4 servings

Vegetable and Bean Paella

I love paella! It's a great rice-based creation to use your leftovers, and the variety of flavors in the dish makes for great dining!

There is a charming legend about how paella got its name. The story is that in fifteenth-century Spain during a period of great hardship, families had very little food. So when marriages took place, everyone brought a little food to "add to the pot" for the meal provided by the bride's family.

The offerings were a little rice, a few vegetables, some chicken, or whatever the family could give. The wedding guests would hand over their donation to the bride's parents by saying, "Para ella," which means "for her," meaning "This is for the bride." All the goods were combined into one large pan and everyone ate!

Other stories exist about the origin of the word *paella,* but this one is so lovely that I enjoy thinking about it whenever I make the dish.

Follow this recipe or be creative by adding ingredients that you and your family enjoy. Keep color, texture, and flavors in mind as you consider different food items.

INGREDIENTS

- 3 tablespoons olive oil
- 1 cup finely chopped onion
- 1 cup long- or medium-grain brown rice
- 2 garlic cloves, minced
- 1 teaspoon ground cumin
- 1 can (15 ounces) stewed tomatoes (with juice)
- 1½ cups vegetable broth
- 1 cup Sonoma dried tomato halves, cut into strips
- 1 can (15 ounces) pinto beans, rinsed and drained
- 1 can (15 ounces) red kidney beans, rinsed and drained
- 1 can (15 ounces) chickpeas, rinsed and drained
- 1 cup finely diced zucchini (¼-inch dice)
- 1 cup frozen corn kernels
- Salt to taste
- ¼ cup chopped cilantro leaves
- 2 tablespoons finely diced red bell pepper
- 2 teaspoons seeded and finely diced jalapeño pepper

1. Heat oil in a large skillet over medium heat; sauté onions about 5 minutes or until golden.

2. Reduce heat to medium-low; stir in rice, garlic, and cumin and stir about 1 minute so all ingredients are well blended and start to cook.

3. Add stewed tomatoes, broth, and dried tomatoes; heat to boiling. Stir to make sure all ingredients are well blended; cover and continue to cook over medium-low heat for 15 minutes.

4. Mix beans, chickpeas, zucchini, and corn in bowl. Add to skillet and stir gently to mix well. Reduce heat to low, cover, and cook about 10–15 minutes or until rice is soft.

5. Adjust seasoning with salt before transferring to serving dish; sprinkle with cilantro, bell pepper, and jalapeño just before serving.

Makes 6 servings

Daniel Fast Cabbage Rolls

This recipe is packed with flavor, nutrients, and interest! Serve as a main dish with Kirsten's Favorite Yellow Rice (page 164) and a green salad for an appetizing meal.

INGREDIENTS

- 12 large cabbage leaves (regular or Napa cabbage)
- 2 tablespoons olive oil
- ½ pound mushrooms, sliced
- 1 cup chopped onion
- 1 cup cooked brown rice
- 1 can (15 ounces) small white beans, rinsed and drained
- 1 cup shredded carrot
- 2 tablespoons chopped parsley
- 1 teaspoon crushed oregano
- ½ teaspoon salt
- ¼ teaspoon pepper
- Vegetable oil to prepare baking pan
- 1 can (15 ounces) tomato sauce
- 1 teaspoon Italian herbs

1. Preheat oven to 350 degrees.

2. Bring a large pot of water to boil; cook cabbage leaves, a few at a time, for about 2 minutes or until softened. Drain and cool.

3. Heat oil over medium heat in a large skillet; sauté mushroom and onion until tender.

4. Add rice, beans, carrot, parsley, oregano, salt, and pepper; stir gently until well blended.

5. Prepare a shallow 2-quart baking dish by brushing with vegetable oil.

6. Spoon mixture onto individual cabbage leaves; roll up and place seam-side down in baking dish.

7. Cover with foil and bake at 350 degrees for 30 minutes.

8. Heat tomato sauce and Italian herbs in small saucepan, stirring often to prevent sticking.

9. Serve cabbage rolls with heated sauce.

Makes 6 servings

Tip: This is one of those meals that includes a few steps during preparation. Consider using meal preparation time to pray, memorize verses, meditate on Scripture, or listen to audio teaching. You'll find the time passing quickly, the experience enriching, and the whole event very rewarding!

Curried Vegetables with Tofu

Enjoy this great meal that's full of nutrition, colors, flavors, and textures! The tofu adds lots of protein to this main dish.

INGREDIENTS

- 2 tablespoons coconut oil
- 1 red onion, cut into thick slices
- 3 cloves garlic, minced
- 12 grape tomatoes, halved
- 2 scallions cut into ¼-inch diagonal slices
- 2 carrots, peeled and cut into ¼-inch diagonal slices
- 2 golden beets, peeled and cut into ¼-inch dice
- 1 block firm tofu, cut into 1-inch cubes
- 2 teaspoons curry powder
- ½ teaspoon crushed red pepper flakes
- 1 jalapeño pepper, finely chopped (optional)
- Salt and pepper to taste
- 1 small zucchini, cut into ½-inch diagonal slices
- 1 can (14 ounces) unsweetened coconut milk
- ¼ cup water
- 1 package (3 ounces) Enoki mushrooms, trimmed and separated into small bundles

- 1 tablespoon freshly squeezed lime juice
- ¼ cup coarsely chopped cilantro
- 3 cups hot cooked brown rice

1. Heat the oil in a large, deep skillet over medium heat; add the onion, garlic, tomatoes, scallions, carrots, and beets and sauté for 3–5 minutes or until the vegetables begin to soften.

2. Add the tofu, curry powder, red pepper flakes, jalapeño pepper, salt, and pepper and stir to coat the vegetables with the oil and spices. Cover and cook for 15 minutes, stirring occasionally until the onions soften and the vegetables release some of their juices.

3. Stir in the zucchini, coconut milk, water, mushrooms, and lime juice. Cover and continue cooking for 10 minutes, stirring occasionally, until the beets are just tender. Stir in the cilantro.

4. Place the rice in the center of a large serving bowl. Spoon the curried vegetables, tofu, and juices around the rice.

Makes 6 servings

Jalapeño Safety!

Until I had my hands flaming after cutting jalapeño peppers, I never looked for a way to protect them from the fiery pepper oil. Then it happened, and believe me, it's no fun! The oil soaks into the skin and doesn't wash off! So now I protect my hands with polyethylene food prep gloves when cooking with fresh jalapeños. This keeps the oil from penetrating the skin, which can be very painful.

Moo Shu Vegetables

Pork is usually the protein ingredient found in this main dish originating in northern China, but this vegetarian variety works well on the Daniel Fast as a great addition to your meal plans. Serve with whole wheat Chapatis or Indian Flatbread (see page 198).

INGREDIENTS

- 2 teaspoons sesame oil
- 3 scallions, thinly sliced
- 3 cups thinly sliced bok choy
- 1 red bell pepper, thinly sliced
- 2 carrots, thinly sliced
- ¾ cup thinly sliced mushroom

- ¾ cup bean sprouts
- 1 block tofu, crumbled
- 3 teaspoons grated fresh ginger
- 2 cloves garlic, minced
- 2 tablespoons tamari or soy sauce
- 1 recipe homemade Hoisin Sauce (see next recipe)
- 6 chapatis

1. Heat sesame oil in a wok or large skillet over medium-high heat; add scallions, bok choy, red bell pepper, carrots, and mushroom; stir-fry vegetables 3–4 minutes until crisp tender.

2. Add sprouts, tofu, ginger, and garlic and continue cooking 2–3 minutes until sprouts are soft. Stir in tamari sauce.

3. To serve, drizzle a spoonful of hoisin sauce across the center of a chapati. Top with a generous helping of vegetables and roll up burrito style.

Makes 6 servings

Hoisin Sauce

Here is the sauce for your Moo Shu Vegetables. You may choose to make it in a larger batch and then refrigerate it for another meal.

INGREDIENTS

- 4 tablespoons soy sauce
- 2 tablespoons 100 percent creamy peanut butter or black bean paste
- 1 tablespoon apple juice concentrate
- 2 teaspoons white vinegar
- ⅛ teaspoon garlic powder
- 2 teaspoons sesame oil
- 20 drops Chinese hot sauce
- ⅛ teaspoon freshly ground black pepper

1. Place all ingredients in a mixing bowl and blend well.

2. Serve with Moo Shu Vegetables with chapatis. Store leftover sauce in an airtight container in the refrigerator.

Makes 4 condiment servings

New Indian Stuffed Peppers

I think peppers make the greatest little packages for the main dish at lunch or dinner. They are colorful, compact, nice to look at, and easy to serve! This recipe has an Indian kick to it, and if you like richly flavorful food, this will be a winner at your table.

INGREDIENTS

- 2 large potatoes, peeled, boiled, and mashed
- 1½ cups spinach, chopped (I like using the frozen, bagged variety; just thaw it first.)
- 1½ cups cooked brown rice
- 3 tablespoons grated fresh ginger (if you want lots of flavor, don't peel)
- 1 tablespoon plus 1 teaspoon garam masala*
- ¼ teaspoon red chili flakes
- 1 teaspoon salt
- 4 sweet bell peppers, mix of red, yellow, orange, and green

1. Preheat oven to 425 degrees.

2. Place the mashed potatoes, spinach, rice, ginger, garam masala, chili flakes, and salt in a large bowl and mix well.

3. Wash the peppers and cut off the tops, removing the stems. Then scrape out the seeds and the rib membranes.

4. Fill each pepper with one-quarter of the potato-spinach-rice mixture, mounding if necessary.

5. Place the peppers in a baking dish and bake for 40 to 45 minutes or until the peppers are softened.

6. Serve hot on individual dining plates.

Makes 4 servings

*Garam masala is a blend of several spices and is available in most supermarkets. You may need to look for it in the natural foods or the bulk foods section with the teas and spices. If you can't find it, check your local health food store. You can also make your own. I've included a simple recipe on page 218.

New Black Bean and Brown Rice Stuffed Peppers

Peggy Lunde of Costa Mesa, California, should open a restaurant and serve her fabulous recipes! I met Peggy on Facebook, where she frequently contributed recipes on the Daniel Fast fan page. This is one of her favorites—and mine too!

I also was touched to hear how the Lord ministered to Peggy during her recent Daniel Fast: "Susan, your book became my template for the Daniel Fast my husband and I did together. I carved out a time each day to sit quietly and remove myself from the world's routine. I read the Bible and devotionals—and journeyed with new eyes. My aim was to seek a greater purpose to use my gifts in a new church community. My passion for good healthy food was rekindled! I created Daniel Fast recipes to keep us nourished as we focused our attention toward specific purposes, attitudes, and most importantly on our Lord."

INGREDIENTS

- 2 cups cooked black beans, rinsed and drained
- 1 cup cooked brown rice
- ½ tablespoon canola oil
- ½ medium red onion, chopped
- 2 cloves garlic, minced
- 1 jalapeño pepper, seeded and finely minced (to taste)
- ½ teaspoon ground cumin
- Kosher salt and freshly ground pepper
- 6–8 black olives, chopped
- 2 large red bell peppers, cut in half lengthwise; seeds and stems removed
- 2 cups 100 percent vegetable or tomato juice
- ¼ cup chopped fresh cilantro

1. Combine beans and brown rice in a medium bowl and set aside.

2. In a small skillet heat the oil over medium-high heat and sauté the onion, garlic, and jalapeño pepper until softened; add the cumin and cook 30 seconds longer; season with a pinch of salt and pepper.

3. Add the sautéed vegetables to bean-rice mixture; stir in chopped olives.

4. Divide the bean mixture between the four pepper halves; place the peppers in a heavy bottomed saucepan where they will fit snugly; pour juice around peppers to cover halfway.

5. Place a tight-fitting lid over the peppers and simmer for 45 minutes or until peppers are tender and the sauce has thickened slightly. Baste the top of the peppers occasionally to keep the filling moist.

6. Serve garnished with chopped cilantro; consider serving this main dish with grilled zucchini and guacamole, all presented on a large platter covered with lettuce leaves.

Makes 4 servings

New Daniel Fast Shepherd's Pie

Serve this piping hot meal with a simple, lightly dressed green salad, and you have a meal your family will enjoy! Share the name of this meal with the other members at the table and talk about our Good Shepherd and His great love for each one gathered together for this meal. If you have children, encourage each of them to share two or three character qualities of their Shepherd, Jesus.

INGREDIENTS
- 2 tablespoons vegetable oil (not necessary if using a Crock-Pot)
- 1 onion, chopped
- 3–4 cloves garlic, minced
- 2 stalks celery, diced
- 2 cups chopped carrots
- 4–5 potatoes, peeled and cut into small chunks
- 1 can (about 15 ounces) garbanzo beans
- 1 bay leaf
- 1 can (about 15 ounces) stewed tomatoes
- 1 large can (about 28 ounces) tomato sauce
- Salt and pepper to taste

Mashed Potato Topping
- 6 small potatoes, peeled and cut into 2-inch pieces
- 2 tablespoons olive oil
- ½ small onion, chopped
- 2 cloves garlic, peeled and minced
- ½ cup unsweetened soy or rice milk
- ½ cup vegetable broth
- Salt and pepper to taste
- Paprika

1. You may want to make the stew portion of this meal in your slow cooker. Just add all the ingredients and cook according to the manufacturer's directions (usually on high for 6 to 12 hours).

2. To prepare on the stove top, heat the oil in a large soup pot over medium heat. Add the onion and garlic, then sauté for 3 to 4 minutes. Add the celery and carrot, and sauté for 3 to 4 more minutes (add a little water to prevent scorching).

3. Add the potatoes, garbanzo beans, bay leaf, stewed tomatoes, and tomato sauce; bring to a simmer and cook until the vegetables are softened, about 30 minutes.

4. Adjust seasoning with salt and pepper.

5. While the stew is cooking, begin preparing the mashed potato topping by boiling potatoes.

6. Heat the oil in a large skillet over medium heat and sauté the onion and garlic until softened.

7. Slowly add the soy or rice milk and vegetable broth, heating just to a boil.

8. When the potatoes are cooked, drain them and return them to the pot; pour the soy milk and vegetable broth mixture into the pot and mash the potatoes until smooth; season with salt and pepper.

9. When the stew is cooked, place the mixture in a large casserole dish. Spoon the mashed potato mixture evenly over the top; sprinkle with paprika.

10. Heat the oven broiler; place the casserole in the oven about 6 to 8 inches from the heat; broil until browned. Serve hot.

Makes 6 servings

New Fast Food Spaghetti Dinner

Here is a fast and easy recipe to prepare for your family on those evenings when time is short and tummies are empty! Serve this hot dinner with a crispy green salad.

INGREDIENTS

- 1 pound uncooked whole grain spaghetti
- 2 cups peeled, chopped, seeded tomato (about 5 medium tomatoes)
- 1 cup crumbled faux feta cheese (see recipe on page 220)
- ⅓ cup chopped, pitted kalamata olives
- ¼ cup capers

- 1½ tablespoons extra-virgin olive oil
- ¾ teaspoon salt
- ½ teaspoon black pepper
- 4 garlic cloves, minced

1. Quickly peel tomatoes by plunging them into the boiling pasta water (before adding the pasta) for 20 seconds; remove with a slotted spoon and quickly slip off the skins while rinsing under cold water.

2. Cook pasta according to package directions, omitting salt and fat. Drain.

3. Combine tomato and remaining ingredients in a large bowl. Add pasta, and toss well to combine. Serve immediately.

Makes 6 servings

New Quinoa and Veggie Bake

Quinoa is a grain-like food, but it's actually a seed that is distantly related to beets and spinach. The seed is packed with protein and fiber. Quinoa's greatest benefit is that it contains all the amino acids necessary to make it a complete protein and is a great alternative for meat. Add colorful veggies and you can't go wrong with this meal.

INGREDIENTS

- 1 cup quinoa
- ¼ cup raisins
- ¼ cup raw sunflower seeds
- 2 bay leaves
- 2 tablespoons olive oil
- 1 cup celery, diced
- 2 medium carrots, diced
- 2 small zucchini, diced
- 1 teaspoon ground coriander
- Pinch cayenne pepper
- ½ teaspoon dried ginger
- ½ teaspoon ground cinnamon
- ½ teaspoon ground cumin
- ½ teaspoon salt
- Freshly ground black pepper

- 1½–1¾ cups boiling water or vegetable broth (use smaller amount for slow cooker or Crock-Pot)
- ¼ cup minced parsley or cilantro for garnish

1. Soak the quinoa for about an hour, then rinse until the water runs clear using a fine-mesh strainer; drain.
2. Preheat the oven to 350 degrees.
3. Heat the olive oil in a large skillet over medium heat; add the celery and sauté until it starts to become transparent; add the carrots and cook for 5 more minutes; add the zucchini and cook for about one more minute.
4. Add the coriander, cayenne pepper, ginger, cinnamon, cumin, salt, and pepper, adjusting the seasoning to your liking. Add the quinoa, raisins, sunflower seeds, and bay leaves; stir until integrated and continue cooking until vegetables are tender, about 3 more minutes.
5. Pour the vegetable and quinoa mixture into a 3- to 4-quart covered casserole dish; add the boiling water or broth; cover.
6. Bake for about 20 minutes or until all the water is absorbed.
7. Remove bay leaves.
8. Garnish with minced fresh parsley or cilantro before serving.

Makes 6 servings

New Stir-Fried Vegetables with Quinoa

I like making this recipe whether I'm fasting or not! It's packed with nutrition, flavor, and color. The dish is easy to double and save for lunches or future meals. It also can be served at room temperature, so leftovers (or "repurposed meals," as my daughter calls them) make a great choice for packed lunches.

INGREDIENTS

- ½ pound firm tofu, drained and sliced about ½-inch thick
- 2 cups broccoli florets
- Salt and pepper to taste
- 1 tablespoon soy sauce
- 1 tablespoon fish sauce (or soy sauce)
- 2 teaspoons sesame oil
- 1 tablespoon minced garlic
- 1 tablespoon minced ginger
- 2 tablespoons canola oil

- 1 stalk celery, chopped
- 1 medium red bell pepper, cut in thin strips
- ¾ pound napa cabbage, cut in 1-inch lengths
- 1 bunch green onions, sliced thin
- 5 cups cooked quinoa (1⅓ cups uncooked)

1. Place the tofu slices between two paper towels.

2. Bring a pot of water to a boil; meanwhile, dice tofu into ½-inch pieces. Add broccoli to boiling water for 1 minute. Transfer immediately to a bowl of ice water. Drain and dry.

3. Combine the soy sauce, fish sauce, and sesame oil in a small bowl. Combine the garlic and ginger in another small bowl.

4. Heat a flat-bottomed wok or skillet over high heat until a drop of water evaporates a second or two after being added to the pan. Coat bottom and sides of wok or skillet with a tablespoon of the oil.

5. Add the tofu. Reduce heat to medium and stir-fry 1 to 2 minutes until it begins to brown. Add the garlic and ginger and stir-fry for no more than 10 seconds. Add the celery, pepper, and napa cabbage and stir-fry for 1 minute. Add the broccoli and stir-fry for 1 minute.

6. Swirl in the remaining oil, and add the green onions, quinoa, and soy sauce mixture. Stir-fry for about 1 minute until heated through.

Makes 4 servings

Soups and Stews

Soups and stews are the mainstay for the Daniel Fast lunch and dinner meals. Most of the recipes are easy and quick to prepare, and they are full of nutrition, flavor, and goodness. I find it very helpful to double the recipes so I can save one in the freezer for a later meal. I also freeze single servings of the soups and stews to use for lunches.

You can follow the recipes in this section as written or adjust them with additional ingredients that you and your family members enjoy.

By the way, do you know that eating soup for meals can also serve as a weight-loss strategy? Soup takes longer to eat and contains more water than dense foods. Our bodies are equipped with a signaling system that tells the brain when we've consumed enough food but it takes about 20 minutes for that message to travel. So when we eat slowly, we allow our God-created system the time it needs to function well. When we consume our food too quickly, we are overriding the system and we consume too many calories. Soup can often satisfy our "dining needs" while also allowing our bodies to function as God intended.

When we habitually overeat, our senses can become "deaf" to the signals sent by the brain telling us we've had enough and to stop eating. The Daniel Fast can help restore our bodies' built-in controls.

> **Tip:** An immersion blender is a great tool to have for making these soup recipes. Many of the recipes instruct cooks to liquefy the soups using a blender or a food processor, but this can be a messy and dangerous process if you are transferring boiling-hot liquids from the pan to the blender. An immersion blender is a great electric tool that is like a blender on a stick! You just insert the end of the blender into your soup and turn it on. Allow it to blend as long as you desire (I prefer to leave some beans whole in my black bean soup), then turn off the device, remove it from your soup, and quickly clean it by running it briefly in plain or soapy water and then rinsing. Mine came with a blending beaker and lid that is great for making smoothies.

Quick Slow Cooker Veggie Soup

This is a great recipe that you can assemble before leaving home and have ready to eat when you return. Serve the soup with homemade flatbread or crackers and a green salad for a nutritious and flavorful meal.

INGREDIENTS

- 2 cans (15 ounces each) diced or crushed tomatoes, with juice
- 1 small can (6 ounces) tomato paste
- 1 can (15 ounces) tomato sauce
- 1 can (15 ounces) yellow corn, drained
- 1 can (15 ounces) green beans, drained
- 1 can (15 ounces) potatoes, drained
- 1 can (15 ounces) peas, drained
- 1 can (15 ounces) sliced carrots, drained
- 2 medium onions, diced
- 1 clove garlic, minced
- 1 tablespoon Italian herbs
- 4–5 bay leaves
- Salt and freshly ground pepper to taste

1. Gently combine the tomatoes, tomato paste, tomato sauce, corn, beans, potatoes, peas, carrots, onions, garlic, Italian herbs, and bay leaves in a large slow cooker or soup pot.

2. If necessary, add water to cover the ingredients; cook in the slow cooker for 3–4 hours, or simmer on the stove top in soup pot.

3. Adjust seasoning with salt and pepper before serving.

Makes 4–6 servings

Golden Carrot Soup

Sweet carrots make a delicious soup that the whole family will enjoy. This soup also freezes well. Once the soup is cool, ladle servings into ziplock bags and lay flat in your freezer, taking out later for lunches or other meals.

INGREDIENTS

- 2 tablespoons olive oil
- 1 large onion, chopped
- 3 stalks celery, chopped
- 2 teaspoons chopped garlic
- 4 cups sliced carrots
- 1 teaspoon Italian herbs
- 1 teaspoon dried basil
- 1 quart vegetable broth
- 1 teaspoon salt
- ½ teaspoon freshly ground black pepper
- Italian parsley for garnish

1. Heat the olive oil in a large pot over medium heat; add the onion, celery, garlic, carrots, Italian herbs, and basil; sauté for about 10 minutes.

2. Pour in the vegetable broth, cover, and adjust heat to simmer for about 25 minutes or until the carrots are tender.

3. To liquefy the soup, pour half of the hot liquid into a blender and blend until smooth. Repeat with the remaining soup. Or use a handheld emulsifier in the same cooking pot.

4. Adjust seasoning with salt and pepper, ladle into individual bowls, garnish, and serve.

Makes 6 servings

Tuscan Villa Bean Soup

I love this soup recipe because it really is brimming with Tuscan flavors and textures. The flavors are as rich as the colors. Add a colorful dinner salad, and you will have an exquisite meal.

INGREDIENTS

- 1 tablespoon olive oil
- 1 cup chopped onion
- ½ cup sliced celery
- 3 cloves garlic, minced
- 1 tablespoon whole wheat pastry flour
- 1 teaspoon dried rosemary leaves
- ¼ teaspoon dried thyme leaves
- 2 bay leaves
- 1 whole clove
- ¼ teaspoon pepper
- 4 cans (15 ounces each) vegetable broth
- 1 can (15 ounces) green baby lima beans, drained and rinsed
- 1 can (15 ounces) chickpeas, drained and rinsed
- 1 can (15 ounces) red beans, drained and rinsed
- 2 tablespoons tomato paste
- 1½ cups cooked barley
- 1 large potato, unpeeled, cut into ½-inch pieces
- 1 cup sliced carrots
- 1 cup packed chopped spinach leaves

1. Heat oil in a large soup pot over medium heat; sauté onions, celery, and garlic for 2–3 minutes; stir in flour, herbs, and pepper and sauté 2–3 minutes or until onions are tender.

2. Add vegetable broth, beans, and tomato paste to pot; heat to boiling, stirring to prevent sticking.

3. Reduce heat and simmer, uncovered, for 10 to 15 minutes.

4. Add barley, potato, carrots, and spinach and simmer 10 more minutes until all ingredients are well heated.

5. Discard bay leaves before serving.

Makes 6 servings

Tomato Paste in a Tube

I used to open a can of tomato paste when a recipe called for just a couple of tablespoons of the ingredient. Then I would store the remainder in an airtight container and forget about it until I cleaned the fridge a couple of weeks later! Aargh! That was until I discovered tomato paste in a tube. It's more expensive, but in the long run it saves a lot with the spared waste! You can find the tomato paste in a tube near the canned variety in larger supermarkets.

Classic Navy Bean Soup the Daniel Fast Way

My mother used to make navy bean soup when I was growing up, but she always added a ham bone to the recipe. This Daniel Fast version is also tasty, and keeps up to a week in the refrigerator, plus it freezes well. Serve a bowl of this hearty soup with a simple salad and Indian Flatbread (page 198) for a delicious meal.

INGREDIENTS

- 1 pound dried navy beans, rinsed and sorted
- 6 cups vegetable broth
- 4 cups water
- 1 yellow onion, finely chopped
- 2 stalks celery, chipped
- 1 carrot, diced
- 4 cloves garlic, minced
- 1 bay leaf
- 3 tablespoons tomato paste
- 1½ teaspoons salt
- ½ teaspoon freshly ground black pepper
- ¼ cup chopped Italian parsley
- ¼ cup finely chopped Italian parsley for garnish

1. Soak the dried beans overnight or for at least 8 hours by placing them in a large pot or bowl with enough water to cover by about 2 inches.

2. Drain and rinse the beans and then place them in a large pot with vegetable broth, water, onion, celery, carrot, garlic, and bay leaf.

3. Bring to a boil and then reduce heat to medium-low. Partially cover and adjust the heat to gently simmer for about 1 hour, or until beans are almost tender.

4. Add tomato paste and salt and continue to cook in partially covered pot until beans are tender, about 30–45 minutes.

5. Remove the bay leaf. Puree half the mixture using a blender, food processor, or immersion blender and add back to the bean pot. Stir in pepper and parsley; reheat to serving temperature and adjust seasoning with salt and pepper.

6. Serve in individual soup bowls and garnish with finely chopped parsley.

Makes 8 servings

Are the Beans Done?

Be sure to sample beans from several places in the cooking pot because they cook at different temperatures. Also, stir your pot a few times to assure even cooking.

Basic Black Bean Soup

This recipe is an excellent choice for lunch or dinner and it freezes well for future meals. I usually make it with canned beans because they are so quick and easy. But you can also use cooked dried beans if you prefer. If you start making a lot of thick soups, you might want to invest in an immersion blender to make your job quicker and cleanup easier.

INGREDIENTS

- 1 tablespoon olive oil
- ¾ cup finely chopped onion
- 1 teaspoon minced garlic
- ¾ cup finely chopped celery
- 2 teaspoons finely chopped jalapeño pepper (use precaution when handling)
- 2 cans (15 ounces each) black beans, rinsed and drained
- 1 can (15 ounces) diced tomatoes, including liquid
- 2 cups water
- 1 teaspoon ground cumin
- Salt, freshly ground black pepper, and red pepper flakes to taste

1. Heat oil in sauté pan over medium heat; add onion and garlic and sauté for 2 minutes.

2. Add celery and jalapeño pepper and sweat for 1 to 2 minutes. Remove from heat and set aside.

3. Place 1 can black beans, half the diced tomatoes, and all the water in a large saucepan (if using immersion blender) or blender. Puree until smooth.

4. Combine the puree, the remaining beans, and tomatoes with the onion, garlic, celery, and jalapeño in the large saucepan. Stir in cumin and then season with salt, pepper, and red pepper flakes as desired.

5. Cover pot and simmer over medium heat until well heated; reduce heat to low and adjust the lid to release steam while simmering for 20 minutes. Serve hot.

Makes 6 servings

Zesty Black Bean Soup with Chipotle Chiles

Dried beans tend to cook unevenly, so be sure to taste several beans to determine their doneness in step 1. Prepare the soup ingredients while the beans simmer and the garnishes while the soup simmers. You don't need to offer all of the garnishes, but choose a couple; garnishes add not only flavor but texture and color as well. Leftover soup can be refrigerated in an airtight container for 3 or 4 days; reheat it in a saucepan over medium heat until hot, stirring in additional vegetable broth if it has thickened beyond your liking. The addition of chipotle chiles in adobo—jalapeños packed in a seasoned tomato-vinegar sauce—makes this a spicier, smokier variation of Black Bean Soup.

INGREDIENTS

- 2 cups dried black beans, picked over, soaked overnight, and rinsed
- 2 bay leaves
- 5 cups water
- 1 teaspoon salt
- 3 tablespoons olive oil
- 3 cups finely chopped onion
- ½ cup finely chopped carrot
- 1 cup finely chopped celery
- ½ teaspoon salt
- 5–6 medium cloves garlic, minced
- 1½ tablespoons ground cumin
- 1 tablespoon Chipotle Chiles in Adobo Sauce (see the next recipe)
- 2 teaspoons adobo sauce
- 6 cups vegetable broth
- 2 tablespoons cornstarch
- 2 tablespoons water
- 2 tablespoons lime juice, from 1–2 limes

Garnishes

- lime wedges
- minced fresh cilantro leaves
- red onion, finely diced
- avocado, diced medium

1. **Cook the beans:** Place beans, bay leaves, and water in large saucepan with tight-fitting lid. Bring to boil over medium-high heat; using large spoon, skim scum as it rises to surface. Stir in salt, reduce heat to low, cover, and simmer briskly until beans are tender, 1¼ to 1½ hours (if necessary, add another cup of water and continue to simmer until beans are tender); do not drain beans. Discard bay leaves.

2. **Cook the soup:** Heat the oil in large soup pot over medium-high heat; add onion, carrot, celery, and salt; sauté while stirring occasionally, about 12–15 minutes or until vegetables are soft and lightly browned. Reduce heat to medium-low; add garlic and cumin and continue to cook until fragrant, about 3 minutes. Stir in the beans, the bean cooking liquid, chipotle chiles, adobo sauce, and vegetable broth. Increase heat to medium-high and bring to boil; reduce heat to low and simmer, uncovered, stirring occasionally for about 30 minutes while flavors blend.

3. **Finishing:** Ladle about 1½ cups beans and 2 cups liquid into food processor or blender, process until smooth, and return to pot (you can also use an immersible blender). Stir together cornstarch and water in small bowl until combined, then gradually stir about half of cornstarch mixture into soup; bring to boil over medium-high heat to thicken soup, stirring occasionally. Adjust the thickening to your liking by adding more of the cornstarch mixture. Remove the pot from the heat, and stir in lime juice before ladling soup into bowls; serve immediately, and offer garnishes separately.

Makes 6 servings

Chipotle Chiles in Adobo Sauce

- 3 cups water
- ½ onion, cut in ½-inch slices
- 5 tablespoons cider vinegar
- 2 cloves garlic, sliced
- ¼ cup tomato sauce
- 1 teaspoon apple juice concentrate
- ¼ teaspoon salt
- 7–10 medium-size dried chipotle chiles, stemmed and slit lengthwise

1. Place all the ingredients in a medium-size saucepan and heat over medium-high heat; bring to a boil.

2. Reduce heat to low, cover pan, and simmer for 60–90 minutes or until the chiles are soft and the liquid is reduced to about 1 cup.

Makes 7–10 chiles

Butternut Curry Soup

Sprinkle lightly toasted pumpkin seeds over each bowl of soup for a nice textural contrast.

INGREDIENTS

- 1 large butternut squash, peeled, seeds removed, cut into 1-inch cubes
- ¼ cup chopped green onions
- 2 tablespoons curry powder
- 3 tablespoons olive oil
- Salt and pepper to taste
- 1 vegetable bouillon cube dissolved in 2 cups of hot water

1. In a medium-size saucepan, boil the squash until tender.

2. Drain most of the water, leaving an inch remaining in the saucepan.

3. Use a potato masher or immersion blender to mix the squash and water until smooth.

4. Stir in green onions, curry, and oil. Season with salt and pepper to taste.

5. Add the bouillon broth in small amounts to reach desired consistency.

6. Simmer for 15 minutes and serve hot.

Makes 4 servings

Plentiful Vegetable Soup

I like to make a big pot of this soup and serve it for dinner, and then serve the leftovers for lunches. It refrigerates well for 2–3 days and heats quickly on top of the stove or in the microwave.

INGREDIENTS

- 2 tablespoons olive oil
- 3 large carrots, peeled and diced into ¾-inch pieces
- 2 large parsnips, peeled and diced into ½-inch pieces
- 2 small onions, peeled and diced into ½-inch pieces

- 6 cloves garlic, minced
- 8 cups vegetable broth
- 2 medium russet potatoes, peeled and diced into 1-inch pieces
- 2 teaspoons minced fresh thyme leaves
- 1 sprig fresh rosemary
- 1 bay leaf
- 2 cups fresh spinach, stemmed and chopped
- 1 can (15 ounces) cannellini beans, drained and rinsed (you can also use kidney beans)
- 1 package (10 ounces) frozen baby lima beans or peas
- 1 tablespoon balsamic vinegar
- Salt and freshly ground black pepper

1. Heat the oil in large soup pot over medium-high heat. Add the carrots, parsnips, and onions and cook until lightly browned and softened, 5–7 minutes.

2. Add the garlic and cook until fragrant, about 30 seconds. Add the vegetable broth, potatoes, thyme, rosemary, and bay leaf; bring to a boil and then reduce heat to low. Cover and continue to simmer until vegetables are soft, about 15 minutes.

3. Remove and discard the rosemary and bay leaf. Transfer 3 cups of the solids and 1 cup of the broth to a blender and puree until smooth.

4. Add the puree back to the soup pot before adding the spinach, cannellini beans, and lima beans; cook over medium heat until spinach is tender and beans are heated through, about 8 minutes.

5. Stir in 1 tablespoon vinegar and season with salt and pepper to taste. Serve, passing extra oil and vinegar at table.

Makes 6–8 servings

Moroccan Vegetarian Stew

A trick to curbing your appetite is to make sure the food you serve is satisfying. One of the best ways to do that is to make recipes that are rich in flavor. Moroccan food fits this bill! It's not only packed with flavor, but the colors and textures make this an attractive dish.

INGREDIENTS

- 2 tablespoons olive oil
- 1 medium yellow onion, chopped

- 4 cloves garlic, minced
- 2 teaspoons ground cumin
- 1 cinnamon stick
- Salt and freshly ground black pepper
- 1 pound butternut squash, diced into 1-inch pieces
- ¾ pound red potatoes, diced into 1-inch pieces
- 2 cups vegetable broth
- 2 cups canned chickpeas, drained
- 1 can (14 ounces) diced tomatoes, including liquid
- Pinch of saffron threads, optional
- 1 tablespoon lemon zest
- 1 cup Greek green olives
- 6 cups steamed whole wheat couscous, for serving
- Fresh cilantro leaves, roughly chopped, for garnish
- Toasted slivered almonds, for garnish

1. Heat the olive oil over medium heat in a 3- to 4-quart Dutch oven or soup pan with a tight-fitting lid. Add onion, garlic, cumin, and cinnamon; season with salt and freshly ground black pepper. Cook, stirring occasionally, until the spices are aromatic and the onions are soft and translucent, about 5 minutes.

2. Stir in the squash and potatoes; reseason with salt and freshly ground black pepper if needed; cook until just tender, about 3 minutes.

3. Add the broth, chickpeas, tomatoes, and saffron, if using. Bring the soup to a boil and then reduce the heat to low. Cover and simmer until squash is fork tender, about 10 minutes.

4. Remove the pot from heat and stir in lemon zest and olives.

5. Serve over couscous garnished with cilantro and almonds.

Makes 6 servings

Susan's Vegetarian Chili

I have been making this recipe for more than twenty years and still enjoy it. The chili is quick to make, colorful, and packed with flavor. It keeps well, so consider making a double recipe to serve a couple of times during the week or freeze for later.

INGREDIENTS

- 2 medium-sized green peppers, chopped
- 1 medium-sized yellow onion, chopped

- 2 tablespoons vegetable oil
- 1 zucchini, sliced
- 1 yellow squash, sliced
- 2 tablespoons chili powder
- ¾ teaspoon salt
- ¼ teaspoon ground red pepper
- 2 cups corn kernels (fresh or frozen)
- 2 cans (16 ounces each) tomatoes, including liquid
- 2 cans (16 ounces each) pinto beans, including liquid
- 2 cans (16 ounces each) black beans, including liquid
- 1 can (4 ounces) mild green chilies, including liquid
- 1 can (4 ounces) tomato paste

1. Chop and sauté the peppers and onion in oil. Add the sliced zucchini and yellow squash, chili powder, salt, ground red pepper, and corn kernels.

2. When all the vegetables are cooked but still firm, add the tomatoes, all the beans, the green chilies, and the tomato paste. Stir until just blended.

3. Bring to a boil and then reduce the heat. Let simmer for 20 minutes, stirring occasionally to prevent sticking.

Makes 6 servings

Tip: All beans, both dried and canned, are high in protein, fiber, vitamins, and minerals. If you use canned beans, be sure to read the label to make sure the manufacturer hasn't added sugar. Also, dried beans are often lower in sodium. Plus they're about half the cost of canned beans! If you cook dried beans, consider preparing a large batch and freezing the leftovers in ziplock bags. They'll keep for up to a year in the freezer.

Hats Off to the Cook Chili with Tofu

Chili is a filling meal, and perfect for the Daniel Fast. The tofu packs the main dish with protein and really does seem like ground beef. Double or even triple this recipe so you have some to freeze. Also, spoon single-serving amounts into ziplock bags, freeze flat, and use for later lunches.

INGREDIENTS

Chili Spice Blend

- 2 tablespoons ground chili powder
- 2 teaspoons ground cumin

- 1 teaspoon dried oregano, crumbled
- ½ teaspoon mustard powder
- ¼ teaspoon cinnamon
- ¼ teaspoon ground cloves
- ¼ teaspoon nutmeg
- ¼ teaspoon ground ginger

Chili

- 2 tablespoons olive oil
- 3 yellow onions, minced
- 2 cloves garlic, minced
- 1 green bell pepper, diced
- 2 teaspoons kosher salt
- Chili Spice Blend
- 2 pounds extra firm tofu, drained and crumbled
- 2 large cans (28 ounces each) diced Italian tomatoes with juice
- 2 cubes vegetable bouillon (or 1 tablespoon VegeBase)
- 1 cup water
- 1 can (15 ounces) red kidney beans, including liquid
- 1 can (15 ounces) pinto beans, including liquid
- 1 pound whole wheat spaghetti
- ½ cup finely chopped onion, for serving

1. Mix the Chili Spice Blend in a small bowl and set aside.

2. Heat the olive oil in a large pot or skillet over medium-high heat. Add the onions and garlic; sauté for 5 minutes.

3. Add the green pepper, salt, Chili Spice Blend, and crumbled tofu. Sauté for about 5 minutes, stirring often as the tofu absorbs the flavors. Stir in the tomatoes with juice.

4. Meanwhile, in a small saucepan mix the bouillon with water; heat and stir until dissolved. Add to chili pot and simmer over medium-low heat for up to 2 hours, adding water if necessary. Long simmering allows the flavors to fuse with all ingredients.

5. Gently blend in the kidney beans, pinto beans, and liquids. Heat while cooking the spaghetti.

6. Cook whole wheat spaghetti following package directions.

7. Serve the chili over the spaghetti noodles in separate bowls. Top with onion if desired.

Makes 12 servings

Tex-Mex Chili Pot

This low-calorie high-protein chili is packed with healthy fiber, plus it's quick and easy to prepare. Create this hearty meal in just 30 minutes; add a green salad and sliced fruit, and you have a lovely "fast food" meal. Tex-Mex Chili also freezes well, so it's a great "make ahead" dish.

INGREDIENTS

- 2 tablespoons olive oil
- 1 tablespoon garlic
- 1 leek, chopped (discard tough leaves first)
- 1 tablespoon chili powder
- 1 teaspoon ground cumin
- 1 red bell pepper, diced
- 1 carrot, diced
- 2 zucchinis or yellow squashes, cut in ½-inch cubes
- 4 cups vegetable broth
- 1 can (15 ounces) black beans, rinsed and drained
- 1 can (15 ounces) pinto beans, rinsed and drained
- 1 can (15 ounces) white beans, rinsed and drained
- ¼ cup chopped fresh cilantro

1. Heat olive oil over medium-high heat; add garlic, leek, chili powder, and cumin and sauté for 3 minutes.

2. Add bell pepper, carrot, and zucchini or yellow squash and cook for 5 more minutes.

3. Stir in broth and increase heat to bring to boil. Reduce heat to medium and add rinsed and drained beans. Cook for 10 minutes until well heated.

4. Stir in fresh cilantro and serve.

Makes 8 servings

Lentil Soup

Lentils are becoming more and more popular as people discover their great flavor and nutritional value. You will enjoy this recipe, especially when served with salad and homemade crackers.

INGREDIENTS

- 2 quarts water
- 3 cups lentils, soaked 2–3 hours

- 2 teaspoons salt
- 2 tablespoons olive oil
- 1 large onion, chopped
- 2 stalks celery, chopped
- 3 carrots, sliced
- 2 cloves garlic, minced
- 2 cans (15 ounces each) diced tomatoes with juice
- 2 tablespoons lemon juice
- 2 tablespoons red wine vinegar
- Freshly ground black pepper to taste
- Dried herbs to taste

1. Heat the water in a large pan over medium-high heat; add the lentils, lower the heat, and cook covered for 20 minutes; add salt.

2. While the lentils are cooking, heat oil in large skillet over medium heat; add onion, celery, carrots, and garlic. Sauté until soft, about 10 minutes.

3. Stir the softened vegetable mixture into the lentils. Add tomatoes, lemon juice, and vinegar; season with pepper.

4. Bring to boil, then gently simmer uncovered until lentils are very tender, about 30 minutes. If the soup becomes too thick, add a little water.

5. Before serving, check the seasoning and stir in chopped herbs.

Makes 6–8 servings

Daniel Fast Cabbage Soup

We've all heard of the "cabbage soup diet." Well, this is not it! However, the nutrients and flavors are rich in this recipe and it's quick to make and low in the calorie department.

INGREDIENTS

- ½ cup olive oil
- 1 yellow onion, chopped
- 4–5 cloves garlic, minced
- 1 red bell pepper, diced large
- 4 stalks celery, chopped
- 1 head green cabbage, cored and sliced
- 2 quarts vegetable stock
- 3 carrots, cut into ½-inch pieces
- 2 cups green beans, cut into ½-inch pieces

- 1 can (15 ounces) diced tomatoes, with juice
- 1 cup brown rice
- 2 tablespoons Italian herbs
- Salt and freshly ground black pepper

1. Heat the olive oil in a large soup or stock pan over medium heat; add the onion, garlic, bell pepper, and celery; sauté until the pepper and celery begin to soften.

2. Add the cabbage, vegetable stock, carrots, green beans, diced tomatoes, rice, and Italian herbs. Adjust heat to a simmer level for the soup.

3. Adjust seasoning with the salt and pepper to taste. Simmer for about 40 minutes or until the rice is cooked and the carrots are tender.

4. Adjust seasoning one more time and serve.

Makes 8–10 servings

Split Green Pea Soup

This soup makes a wonderful meal and also freezes well.

INGREDIENTS

- 2 cups dried green split peas (rinse but do not soak)
- 8 cups vegetable broth
- 2 potatoes, diced large
- 2 carrots, sliced
- ½ cabbage, coarsely chopped
- 1 onion, diced
- 2 cloves garlic, minced
- 2 tablespoons olive oil
- 1 teaspoon cumin
- 1 teaspoon sage
- 1 teaspoon thyme
- 3 bay leaves
- Salt and pepper to taste
- Minced Italian parsley for garnish

1. Combine the split peas, vegetable broth, potatoes, carrots, cabbage, onion, garlic, olive oil, cumin, sage, thyme, and bay leaves in a Crock-Pot or slow cooker. Cover and cook on low for at least 4 hours, or until peas are soft.

2. Remove bay leaves and season with salt and pepper.

3. Serve with minced parsley sprinkled on top.

New **Celery Root Soup**

This is a creamy soup with a little punch to it and packed with flavor. The surprising ingredient in this soup is cashew cream, which gives the soup its creamy texture.

INGREDIENTS

- Pinch of salt
- 3 tablespoons extra-virgin olive oil
- 2 medium celery roots, peeled and cut into 1-inch cubes
- 2 stalks celery, chopped
- 1 large white onion, chopped
- 1 garlic clove, finely chopped
- 2 quarts low-sodium vegetable broth
- 1 bay leaf
- 1¼ cups thick cashew cream (see recipe on page 219)
- Salt and freshly ground black pepper
- 1 Braeburn or Fuji apple, diced fine
- 1 bunch of chives, snipped

1. To give your pan a nonstick effect, heat a large stockpot over medium heat; sprinkle the bottom with a pinch of salt and heat for 1 minute. Add the oil and heat for 30 seconds.

2. Add the celery root, celery, onion, and garlic; sauté until soft, 6–10 minutes, stirring often.

3. Add the vegetable broth and bay leaf. After bringing to a boil, reduce the heat and simmer about 30 minutes. Add cashew cream and simmer for another 10 minutes.

4. Use an immersion blender to process soup until smooth; or working in batches, pour soup into a blender, cover with lid, and place a towel on top to prevent soup from erupting; blend on high until soup is smooth.

5. Season the soup with salt and pepper to taste.

6. After ladling soup into bowls, top with a spoonful of diced apple and pinch of chives in the center of each serving.

Makes 6 servings

Bean and Garden Burgers

A lot of people really miss meat on the Daniel Fast. I used to use portobello mushrooms as a meat substitute but they can be expensive! The only garden burgers I've been able to find in the supermarket freezer case include sweeteners or eggs, so that takes them off the list.

Then I found recipes to make my own garden burgers at home. They are so easy, inexpensive, and full of nutrition and flavor. Make them in larger batches and freeze the patties for later use. Just separate them with a sheet of waxed paper and enclose a stack of the patties in a ziplock freezer bag. You can cook them just like beef patties, but at lower temperatures.

EZ Veggie Burgers

After whipping up these little gems, you may find them on your menu several times a week. The beans are much less expensive than ground beef, and the fat content is almost nil. These burgers make a great option for your Daniel Fast meals.

INGREDIENTS

- 1 can (15 ounces) white navy beans, drained
- ¾ cup crushed whole wheat matzo
- ½ cup chopped yellow onion
- 2 cloves garlic, minced
- ¼ cup chopped Italian parsley
- 2 tablespoons olive oil

1. Using a food processor, mix all the ingredients. Pulse only 4 or 5 times.

2. Divide mixture into 4 mounds. Wet hands slightly and make each of the mounds into a patty.

3. Grill or fry the burgers in a lightly oiled nonstick pan for 4 to 5 minutes, turning once.

4. Serve with chapatis or with a sauce.

Makes 4 servings

Basic Bean Burgers

These bean burgers can surely meet your protein needs. Plus they are excellent for main dishes. Serve these burgers with a rice side dish and a green salad, and you are set to go!

INGREDIENTS

- 1 cup TVP (textured vegetable protein) granules, a soy protein product available in most health food stores.
- 1 tablespoon tomato paste or ketchup
- 1 scant cup boiling water
- 1 can (15 ounces) pinto, kidney, or other beans, drained
- ¼ cup crushed whole wheat matzo
- 2 cloves garlic, finely minced
- ½ teaspoon oregano
- 1 tablespoon tamari or soy sauce
- Salt and pepper to taste
- Whole wheat flour for dusting

1. Place TVP and tomato paste in a large bowl. Pour boiling water over the contents and stir; let rest for 10 minutes while TVP is reconstituted.

2. Using a food processor, combine TVP mixture and remaining ingredients except for flour. Pulse until mixture is almost a puree.

3. Dust hands with flour and shape mixture into six burgers. Dust them lightly in flour. Layer the burgers between sheets of waxed paper and refrigerate for at least 1 hour.

4. Cook on a grill covered with foil or in a well-oiled nonstick skillet for about 10 minutes on each side.

Makes 6 servings

Best Veggie Burger

This recipe has a lot of wonderful flavors. The tanginess of Granny Smith apples works well with all the vegetables!

INGREDIENTS

- ¼ pound green beans
- ½ cup cracked wheat
- 1 small zucchini
- 1 small carrot, peeled

- ½ Granny Smith apple, peeled
- ½ cup canned chickpeas, rinsed and drained
- 1 tablespoon onion, minced
- 1 tablespoon sesame tahini or peanut butter
- ½ teaspoon curry powder
- ½ teaspoon chili powder
- ½ teaspoon salt
- Ground black pepper, to taste
- ½ tablespoon canola oil
- ½ cup matzo crumbs

1. Cook green beans in boiling water until tender-crisp. Drain and chop fine.

2. Meanwhile, cook cracked wheat in 1 cup boiling water for 1 minute. Remove from heat and cover.

3. Grate the zucchini, carrot, and apple. Place shreds in a dish towel and squeeze out excess moisture and then combine with chopped beans.

4. Using a food processor, blend chickpeas, onion, tahini, curry powder, chili powder, salt, pepper, and canola oil until smooth. Add to bowl of shredded vegetables and mix again.

5. Drain cracked wheat in a strainer, removing as much of the liquid as possible.

6. Add to bowl with vegetables; mix in matzo crumbs until all ingredients are well blended. Cover and refrigerate for 1 hour.

7. With wet hands, shape into four burgers. Cook 3 minutes on each side on grill or skillet lightly brushed with oil.

Makes 4 servings

Homemade Veggie Burgers

Potatoes make great veggie burgers! Like latkes (potato pancakes), potatoes absorb the flavors they're added to, and they also have a pleasant texture. You can also adjust this recipe's seasonings to your liking.

INGREDIENTS

- 1 cup canned black beans, drained
- 1 carrot, grated
- ½ onion, diced
- 3 medium potatoes, grated
- 4 scallions, chopped
- 1 cup frozen corn, thawed

- Salt and freshly ground black pepper to taste
- 2 tablespoons olive oil for frying

1. Place the beans in a large bowl and mash with a fork or potato masher. Add the carrot, onion, potatoes, scallions, and corn; mix until well combined. Season with salt and pepper.

2. Wet hands and shape the mixture into four patties.

3. Heat about 2 tablespoons of olive oil and cook each patty until the veggie burgers are done, about 3 minutes on each side.

Makes 4 servings

Popeye Burgers

I suppose there are now a couple of generations that don't know Popeye the Sailor. Okay, I'm dating myself! But spinach is the ingredient that gives this recipe the Popeye name. These burgers are very nutritious and easy to make.

INGREDIENTS

- 1 box (10 ounces) frozen chopped spinach, thawed
- 1 large potato, grated
- 1 medium onion, finely chopped
- 1 tablespoon garlic powder
- 1 tablespoon dried chopped onion
- ½ teaspoon paprika
- ½ cup homemade Daniel Fast Ketchup (see page 217)
- ½ cup crushed whole wheat matzo
- ½ cup rolled oats
- ½ cup cornmeal
- 1 teaspoon Spike or another seasoning salt
- 1 teaspoon Dijon mustard

1. Blend all the ingredients thoroughly in a large mixing bowl, adding a little more cornmeal if the mixture is too wet or a little water if the mixture is too dry.

2. Form into thin patties (the thinner the better) and fry in a lightly oiled nonstick pan over medium heat.

3. You can also freeze uncooked patties by layering them between waxed paper or plastic wrap and sealing in a ziplock bag.

Makes about 12 burgers

Spicy Mexican Bean Burgers

Yummy is all I can say to describe these veggie burgers! Serve them with a nice salad or with a beans-and-rice dish.

INGREDIENTS

- 1 can (15 ounces) red kidney beans, drained and mashed
- ½ onion, coarsely chopped
- ½ green pepper, coarsely chopped
- 1 carrot, steamed and mashed
- 2 tablespoons picante sauce or salsa (spicy or mild to your taste)
- 1 cup crushed rice cakes or whole wheat crackers (matzo)
- ½ cup whole wheat flour
- ½ teaspoon salt (or to taste)
- ½ teaspoon black pepper (or to taste)
- Dash chili powder

1. Preheat oven to 450 degrees.

2. Mix all ingredients in a large mixing bowl. Add more flour to create a firmer mixture or more salsa if mixture is too stiff.

3. Form mixture into balls and then into patties.

4. Place the patties on a broiler or oiled baking dish.

5. Bake for 15–20 minutes until firm, brown, and done.

Makes 8 to 10 burgers

Side Dishes

These recipes can be used as side dishes for a main course, or you can serve several of them along with a salad for a complete meal. You'll find a good variety here, and many recipes offer opportunities for your own culinary creativity.

White Beans with Winter Vegetables

While the vegetables in this recipe are technically "winter veggies" and it's great for warming your insides on cold winter days . . . I love making this dish all year round.

INGREDIENTS

- 1 pound dried cannellini beans, rinsed and picked over
- 1 large onion, peeled and halved from top to bottom
- 4 cloves garlic, unpeeled
- 1 bay leaf
- 1 teaspoon salt
- ¼ cup extra-virgin olive oil, plus extra for serving
- 2 carrots, diced medium
- 2 ribs celery, diced medium
- 2 small leeks, white and light green parts, sliced crosswise into ½-inch pieces
- 1 small onion, diced medium
- 3 cloves garlic, minced
- 3 cups coarsely chopped kale leaves
- 3 cups coarsely chopped escarole
- 2 boiling potatoes, diced medium
- 1 can (15 ounces) diced tomatoes, drained
- 1 sprig fresh rosemary
- Salt and freshly ground black pepper
- Italian parsley for garnish

1. Using a large, heavy-bottomed Dutch oven, combine 12 cups water, the beans, onion, unpeeled garlic, bay leaf, and 1 teaspoon salt; bring to a boil over medium-high heat.

2. Cover the soup pot partially and reduce the heat to low; simmer until the beans are almost tender, about 1 hour, stirring occasionally.

3. Remove the pot from the heat and cover; let it stand until beans are tender, about 30 minutes.

4. Drain, reserving cooking liquid; discard the onion, garlic, and bay leaf and then spread the beans in an even layer on baking sheet to cool.

5. Using your same Dutch oven, heat the oil over medium heat; add the carrots, celery, leeks, and diced onion; cook until the vegetables are softened but not browned, about 7 minutes, stirring occasionally.

6. Stir in minced garlic and cook about 30 seconds. Add 9 cups of the reserved bean cooking liquid (add more water if needed), and then stir in the kale and escarole. Increase the heat to medium-high and bring to boil.

7. Cover the pot and then reduce the heat to low and simmer 30 minutes.

8. Add the potatoes and tomatoes, cover and cook until potatoes are tender, about 20 minutes.

9. Now add the cooled beans and rosemary and continue simmering until the beans are well heated, about 5 minutes.

10. Remove the pot from the heat, cover, and let rest for 15 to 20 minutes. Discard the rosemary sprig and season with salt and pepper to taste.

11. To serve, ladle the soup into individual bowls, drizzle each serving with extra-virgin olive oil, and garnish with parsley.

Makes about 10 servings

Green Beans and Tomatoes Italian Style

This Italian recipe uses a simple tomato sauce flavored with onions and garlic as the braising medium. Add the parsley (or basil) at the end of cooking for extra color.

INGREDIENTS

- 2 tablespoons olive oil
- 1 small onion, diced
- 2 small cloves garlic, minced
- 1 cup canned chopped tomato
- 1 pound green beans, stem ends snapped off
- Salt and freshly ground black pepper
- 2 tablespoons fresh parsley leaves, minced

1. Heat oil in large sauté pan over medium heat. Add onion; cook until softened, about 5 minutes.

2. Add garlic and continue cooking another minute. Add tomatoes; simmer until juices thicken slightly, about 5 minutes.

3. Add green beans, ¼ teaspoon salt, and a few grindings of pepper to pan. Stir well, cover, and cook, stirring occasionally, until beans are tender but still offer some resistance to the bite, about 20 minutes. Stir in parsley and adjust seasonings. Serve immediately.

Makes 4 servings

Roasted Asparagus the Roman Way

I'm not sure how often this recipe is eaten in Rome, but it screams with Mediterranean influence. Even if you don't like asparagus, give this recipe a try to see if your taste buds will change your mind. The flavors are delightful, and the colors are appetizing. You may never want to serve asparagus any other way after using this recipe!

INGREDIENTS

- 1 pound asparagus spears, washed and trimmed
- 10 cherry tomatoes, halved
- ½ cup chopped kalamata olives

Herb and Garlic Marinade

- ⅓ cup water
- ⅓ cup vinegar
- ⅓ cup vegetable oil
- 3 cloves garlic, minced
- 1 teaspoon dried thyme
- 1 teaspoon dried Italian-style seasoning
- 1 teaspoon dried rosemary, crushed
- 1 teaspoon salt
- 1 teaspoon ground black pepper

1. Prepare the oven by placing the rack on the highest position and heating the oven to 450 degrees.

2. Whisk together all the marinade ingredients in a small bowl.

3. Place the asparagus on a large rimmed plate or baking dish. Drizzle some of the marinade over the spears until they are well coated. Reserve the remainder of the marinade for other recipes or for salad dressing.

4. Transfer the spears to a heavy-weight rimmed baking sheet. Scatter the tomatoes and the olives over the asparagus and then bake for about 5 to 10 minutes or until the spears are at the tenderness you desire. Be sure to watch them carefully so they don't overcook.

Makes 4 servings

Fast Food Stir-Fry Brown Rice with Vegetables

You can whip up this healthy Daniel Fast meal in less time than it would take to order and wait for the pizza guy to arrive. Plus this dish is packed with great flavors, and it's so good for you. This is also a great way to use leftovers or add ingredients that you especially enjoy.

INGREDIENTS

- 2 tablespoons olive oil, divided
- 1 onion, sliced
- 2 cloves garlic, minced
- 1 package (16 ounces) frozen stir-fry vegetables
- 4 cups cooked brown rice
- Soy sauce to taste
- ¼ cup roasted peanuts

1. Using a wok or large skillet, heat about 2 tablespoons of oil over medium heat; add the sliced onion and garlic; sauté for about 5 minutes or until onion begins to soften.
2. Add the frozen vegetables to the pan; stir and toss as they cook and heat thoroughly.
3. Stir in the brown rice and season with soy sauce to your taste.
4. Continue to cook until everything is thoroughly heated.
5. Just before serving, garnish with roasted peanuts.

Makes 4 servings

Herb-Roasted Sweet Potato Fries

If you do a little research, you will quickly learn that sweet potatoes are so much better for you than the typical variety of potato. These fries are flavorful and fun to eat. They make a great addition to your hearty salads, soups, and stews; or serve them as a snack or appetizer. You may never go back to the "other fries" again!

INGREDIENTS

- 1 pound small sweet potatoes or yams
- 2 teaspoons olive oil
- ½ teaspoon dried thyme
- ½ teaspoon dried rosemary
- ¼ teaspoon salt
- ⅛ teaspoon freshly ground black pepper

1. Preheat the oven to 425 degrees. Coat a heavy-weight rimmed baking sheet, with cooking spray or brush with vegetable oil.

2. Cut each potato in half crosswise. Place the halves cut side down on the cutting board and cut each into 4 wedges.

3. Combine the oil, thyme, rosemary, salt, and pepper in a large bowl. Add the potato wedges and toss to coat well.

4. Transfer the potatoes to the prepared baking sheet, spreading them out in a single layer. Bake for about 35 minutes, tossing 2 or 3 times, until the potatoes are tender and lightly browned.

5. Serve hot.

Makes 4 servings

Mexican-Style Pickled Vegetables

More than 20 years ago, I started traveling in Mexico and staying in a little place right on the Pacific Ocean. I've returned almost every year since and have formed many wonderful friendships with other travelers and with some of the local people. I've also gained a great appreciation for good Mexican food. This recipe is fairly common in Mexico, and the flavors are wonderful. Enjoy!

INGREDIENTS

- ¾ cup extra-virgin olive oil
- 12 cloves garlic, peeled
- 1 yellow onion, peeled and cut into wedges
- 4 carrots, peeled and sliced diagonally
- 1 teaspoon whole black peppercorns
- 1 teaspoon dried thyme
- 1 teaspoon dried oregano
- 1 teaspoon dried marjoram
- 8 bay leaves
- Salt
- 1 head cauliflower, cored and cut into florets
- 4 jalapeño peppers, seeded and chopped (use precaution when handling)
- 1½ cups white vinegar
- 1 cup water
- 3 zucchinis, sliced diagonally
- 1 large jicama, peeled and cut into ¾-inch dice

1. Heat the oil in a large pan or skillet over medium-high heat; add the garlic and onion and sauté for 3 minutes, stirring constantly.

2. Reduce the heat to medium and add the carrots, peppercorns, thyme, oregano, marjoram, and bay leaves. Cover and cook 2 minutes. Season to taste with salt.

3. Add the cauliflower, jalapeño peppers, vinegar, and 1 cup water. Gently blend, cover, and continue to cook over medium heat for 5 minutes.

4. Gently stir in the zucchini and jicama. Cover and cook for about 5 more minutes, just long enough so the vegetables are still crunchy.

5. Discard bay leaves and transfer the mixture to an airtight refrigerator container; chill in the refrigerator for at least 12 hours or up to 1 week.

6. Serve at room temperature as a condiment or appetizer.

Makes 6–8 condiment servings

Tomatoes, Mushrooms, and Herbs with Rice

Here's another yummy dish that's quick to make. Use this recipe as a substantial side dish or main course. You can also substitute the rice with whole wheat pasta for a nice change.

INGREDIENTS

- 3 tablespoons olive oil
- 2–3 cloves garlic, minced
- 3 tablespoons balsamic vinegar
- Salt and freshly ground black pepper
- 1 pound sliced mushrooms
- 3–5 heirloom or Roma tomatoes, diced medium
- 1 cup fresh basil, cut into thin strips
- 4 servings of cooked brown rice or cooked whole wheat pasta (hot for serving)

1. Heat the oil, garlic, vinegar, salt, and pepper in a medium pan over medium heat; add the sliced mushrooms and sauté lightly for 3–4 minutes.

2. Add the tomatoes, and continue cooking until they are slightly cooked and well heated.

3. Add the basil right before you are ready to serve and cook just 1 more minute.

4. To serve, divide the brown rice or whole wheat pasta onto individual plates and then spoon the tomatoes, mushrooms, and herbs over the top. Serve hot.

Makes 4 servings

Mashed Sweet Potatoes

Most of us grew up on mashed potatoes with melted butter or homemade gravy. While the flavor is high, the nutritional value is wanting when compared to the sweet potato. Sweet potatoes are packed with complex carbohydrates, help to maintain blood sugar levels, and are off the charts as an anti-inflammatory vegetable. This recipe is a healthy addition to any meal, and blending in the tofu increases the protein without altering the flavor.

INGREDIENTS
- 2 pounds sweet potatoes; wash and then trim ends off
- 3 tablespoons silken tofu
- 1 tablespoon unsweetened soy milk

1. Preheat the oven to 400 degrees.

2. Place the potatoes in a large oven-proof dish to capture the sugar during baking. Bake the sweet potatoes in their jackets for 40–60 minutes or until tender, depending on the size of the potato.

3. When the potatoes are cool enough, remove the jackets and place the potatoes in a large bowl. Add tofu and soy milk and then mash with a fork or potato masher.

4. Season as desired and serve hot.

Be creative with the seasonings!

1. Add ½ teaspoon cinnamon to bowl, mash sweet potatoes, and serve.

2. Add ½ teaspoon cinnamon, ½ teaspoon nutmeg, and ½ teaspoon vanilla to the bowl; mash sweet potatoes and serve.

3. Before baking the potatoes, cut the top off a whole garlic bulb to expose the top of each clove; place in the same baking dish as the potatoes and drizzle with olive oil. Bake the garlic for about 45 minutes. Squeeze the garlic cloves from the skins and mash. Add to potatoes and blend. Season with chopped chives or Italian parsley.

Makes 4 servings

Stylin' with Green Peas

Heating green peas in a little boiling salted water is the standard (excuse me while I yawn), but with just a spurt of creativity, we can turn the lowly boiled green pea into something to talk about. Follow the basic recipe below and then add your own flair. See ideas below.

INGREDIENTS

- 2 teaspoons olive oil
- 4 cups frozen green peas, thawed and well drained
- Salt and freshly ground black pepper to taste

1. Heat the oil in a large skillet over medium heat. Add the peas and cook for 8 to 10 minutes until the peas are well heated, stirring often.
2. Add salt and freshly ground black pepper to taste.

Now go wild with your own concoction!

1. During the last minute of cooking, add ¼ teaspoon of lemon pepper, 1 teaspoon of lemon zest, and ¼ teaspoon of dried dill to peas. Heat through and adjust seasoning with salt. Serve hot.
2. Add 1–2 tablespoons minced fresh mint to the peas in the last minute of cooking. Season with salt and freshly ground black pepper; garnish with chopped pecans and serve.
3. Before adding the peas to the skillet, add 1 chopped onion and 2 cloves of minced garlic. Sauté for 2 minutes; add peas and cook for 4 more minutes; add 1 cup sliced fresh mushroom and ¼ teaspoon dried thyme, and cook for an additional 2 minutes or until all ingredients are well heated. Season with salt and freshly ground black pepper. Serve hot.
4. Add 8–10 asparagus spears, cut in 1-inch pieces, to the peas when cooking. Just before serving, add 5–6 cherry tomatoes (cut in half). Heat for about 1 more minute. Season to taste with salt and freshly ground black pepper.

Makes 4 servings

New Baked Curried Cauliflower

If you like curry, this is a great recipe and very easy to prepare. The flavors are pleasant, and although the roasting takes some time, the prep is quick and simple.

INGREDIENTS

- 1 large head cauliflower
- 3 tablespoons olive oil
- 1 tablespoon curry powder
- ½ teaspoon salt
- Cooking spray

1. Core cauliflower and break into medium florets; rinse and drain.

2. Preheat oven to 425 degrees.

3. Using a large bowl, whisk together the olive oil, curry powder, and salt.

4. Add the cauliflower to the bowl and toss until each piece is coated with the curry mixture.

5. Coat a baking pan with cooking spray, and then spread the cauliflower on the surface in a single layer. Cover with foil and place in preheated oven.

6. Bake for 20 minutes; remove foil and continue to roast for another 20 minutes or until cauliflower is softened. Serve hot or at room temperature.

Make 4 to 6 servings

New Quinoa with Vegetables

Originating in South America, quinoa is becoming a popular addition to the diets of those who take good care of their health and want to obtain adequate protein from a plant-based meal.

INGREDIENTS

- Cooking spray
- 1 cup quinoa, rinsed
- 2 cups low-sodium vegetable broth
- ¼ cup water
- 1 tablespoon olive oil
- 1 small yellow onion, chopped
- 1 medium sweet red pepper, chopped

- 1 small carrot, chopped
- 1 cup chopped fresh kale
- 2 cloves garlic, minced
- 1 teaspoon dried basil
- ¼ teaspoon freshly ground black pepper

1. Coat a small saucepan with cooking spray; heat over medium heat and then add quinoa. Roast the seeds until golden brown, stirring often.

2. Add broth and water to pan and bring to a boil; reduce heat and simmer uncovered until liquid is absorbed, stirring often.*

3. Meanwhile, heat the olive oil in a large skillet over medium heat; add onion and sauté until softened, about 2 minutes; add bell pepper, carrot, kale, and garlic and sauté for 3 more minutes.

4. Add the basil and black pepper to the mixture; stir in cooked quinoa and serve hot.

*If you've never eaten quinoa, you may be surprised to see little sprouts emerge when it's cooked.

Makes 4 servings

New Cauliflower with Sweet Potatoes and Tomato

This side dish stands out for its great color and flavors. I sometimes double the recipe and serve it for a couple of meals. It's tasty and full of nutrition.

INGREDIENTS

- 2 tablespoons olive oil
- 2 medium onions, chopped
- 1 clove garlic, finely chopped
- 2 tablespoons grated fresh ginger (if you want lots of flavor, don't peel it)
- 1 tablespoon coriander seeds
- 1 tablespoon cumin seeds
- 1 teaspoon turmeric
- 1 teaspoon salt
- 1 large Roma tomato, peeled, seeded, and chopped
- 1 large sweet potato or yam, peeled and cut into 1-inch chunks
- 1 head cauliflower, cut into bite-sized florets
- ¼ cup unsalted cashews, chopped

1. Heat the oil in a large skillet over medium-high heat; add onions, garlic, and ginger, cook for 4 minutes, stirring to keep them from scorching.

2. Mix in the coriander seeds, cumin seeds, turmeric, and salt; toasting the seeds for 15 to 30 seconds.

3. Add the tomato and sweet potato; cook until tender, about 12 to 15 minutes.

4. Add the cauliflower, tossing to combine; cover and steam until the cauliflower is crisp-tender, about 5 to 7 minutes. Top with cashews.

5. Serve hot.

Makes 4 to 6 servings

Rice and Whole Grains

Whole grains are little workhorses for our health. Not only are they packed with healthy nutrients, but they also help lower cholesterol and improve digestion. I eat a whole grain cereal for breakfast almost every morning and also serve rice a few times each week.

You may also have noticed that most stores now sell a selection of whole grain pasta. You'll want to read the labels to make sure the manufacturer hasn't added sweetener as an ingredient. I make my own red sauce, since I have yet to find a prepared sauce that is sweetener-free.

A time-saving strategy I use is to keep steamed brown rice ready all the time. I have a small rice steamer I picked up for less than twenty dollars. It cooks two cups of uncooked rice at one time. I just add the rice with water (two times more rice than water is the usual ratio) and a teaspoon of pepper or soy sauce and leave the rice until the cooker's automatic turn-off switch stops the cooking. The result is four cups of perfectly cooked rice that's ready to eat or save for other meals. I use brown rice in many dishes and also love eating it for breakfast with chopped apples, raisins, and coconut oil.

Kirsten's Favorite Yellow Rice

My daughter Kirsten could eat this for breakfast, lunch, and dinner! The sweetness in the apple and raisins contrasts with the lemon zest and turmeric.

INGREDIENTS

- 4 cups water
- 1 cup chopped sweet apple (no peels—I just eat the peelings while I prepare this dish)
- ½ teaspoon turmeric
- 1 tablespoon salt
- 2 tablespoons canola oil
- 1 cinnamon stick
- 1 cup raisins
- 1 teaspoon lemon zest
- 2 cups long-grain brown rice

1. Heat the water in a large pot over high heat; add the apple, turmeric, salt, canola oil, cinnamon stick, raisins, and lemon zest. Bring to a boil.

2. Stir in rice, reduce heat, cover, and simmer for about 20 minutes or until rice is tender.

3. Remove the cinnamon stick before serving.

Makes about 6 servings

Sweet and Fiery Pineapple Rice

The combination of flavors in this rice side dish keeps your taste buds asking for more! Plus the colors make this look so appetizing.

INGREDIENTS

- 3 cups water
- 1 teaspoon salt
- 1½ cups short-grain brown rice
- 1 jalapeño pepper, seeded and finely chopped (use precautions when handling)
- 1 cup crushed canned pineapple, drained
- ⅓ cup chopped roasted cashew nuts
- ¼ cup chopped fresh cilantro
- Salt and freshly ground black pepper to taste

1. Bring water and salt to a boil over high heat; add the rice and jalapeño pepper; reduce heat to medium, cover, and allow to cook for 20 minutes or until rice is tender.

2. Remove from heat and stir in pineapple, cashews, and cilantro. Adjust seasoning with salt and pepper before serving.

Makes 6 servings

Mexican Rice Pilaf

This is one of my favorite recipes because it's great to serve as a meal and also makes a great leftover dish for lunch the next day.

INGREDIENTS
- 2½ cups water
- 1½ teaspoons salt, divided
- ½ teaspoon freshly ground black pepper
- 1 tablespoon olive oil
- 1 small onion, finely chopped
- 2 jalapeño peppers, stemmed, seeded, and minced (use precaution when handling)
- 1 tablespoon tomato paste
- 2 cloves garlic, minced
- 1½ cups long-grain brown rice
- ¼ cup minced fresh cilantro
- 1 medium tomato, halved, seeded, and diced small
- 1 tablespoon fresh lime juice

1. Heat the water in a small saucepan over medium-high heat. Add 1 teaspoon salt and the ground black pepper; bring to a boil, then reduce heat and cover to keep hot. Set aside for later.

2. Meanwhile, heat the oil over medium-low heat in a large saucepan or skillet; add the onion, chiles, and ½ teaspoon salt and blend. Cover and cook, stirring occasionally, until the onion is softened, 8–10 minutes.

3. Increase the heat to medium and add the tomato paste and garlic. Cook for just 30 seconds or so.

4. Add the brown rice and stir to coat the grains with oil. Cook until the edges of the grains begin to turn translucent, about 3 minutes. Now add the hot water you prepared earlier and bring the mixture to a boil.

5. Reduce the heat to low, cover, and simmer until all the water is absorbed and the rice is cooked, 16–18 minutes.

6. Remove the pot from the heat and sprinkle the mixture with the cilantro and tomato, but do not stir the rice at this point.

7. Lay a clean, folded kitchen towel over the uncovered pot and then place the lid on top. Let the rice stand for 10 minutes.

8. Add the lime juice and gently stir and fluff the rice mixture with a fork; adjust the seasoning with salt and pepper to taste.

Makes 6 servings

Lemony Walnut Rice Pilaf

I love hearing from men and women who end up changing their eating habits after realizing the health benefits of the Daniel Fast. This is one recipe that many people like to keep in their meal plans throughout the year, either for a side dish or even a lunch with a green salad and fruit.

INGREDIENTS

- ½ cup coarsely chopped walnuts
- 2 teaspoons olive oil
- 1 yellow bell pepper, cut in strips
- ½ red onion, cut in strips
- 2 cloves garlic, minced
- 2 cups cooked brown rice
- ¼ cup chopped Italian parsley
- ½ teaspoon lemon zest
- 2 tablespoons lemon juice
- Salt to taste

1. Toast the walnuts by heating them in a skillet over medium-high heat for 3 to 5 minutes, tossing frequently. Set aside to add later.

2. Heat the olive oil in a skillet over medium heat; add bell pepper, onion, and garlic; sauté for about 5 minutes, stirring often. Add the cooked rice and mix well.

3. Stir in nuts, parsley, lemon zest, and lemon juice until all the ingredients are well heated.

4. Season to taste with salt. Serve.

Makes 4 servings

Faux Fried Rice

This recipe takes a little extra prep time, but it's well worth the effort with all the flavors, colors, and great nutrition! Serve this dish with an Asian salad and you have a tasty healthy meal.

INGREDIENTS

- 2 tablespoons olive oil, plus additional amount if necessary as cooking
- 1 package (16 ounces) extra firm tofu, cubed
- 3 tablespoons soy sauce
- 2 tablespoons Chinese mustard
- 2 tablespoons chili paste
- 2 tablespoons sesame oil (available in the Asian foods section of most supermarkets)
- 4 scallions, minced
- 2 carrots, peeled and diced
- 2 cloves garlic, minced
- 3 cups cooked short-grain brown rice
- 1 cup frozen peas, thawed

1. Heat oil in large sauté pan over medium-high heat; add cubed tofu and brown on all sides.

2. Meanwhile, combine soy sauce, Chinese mustard, chili paste, and sesame oil in a medium bowl.

3. When tofu is browned, spoon into soy sauce mixture and set aside.

4. If necessary, add a bit more olive oil to the sauté pan before adding scallions, carrots, and garlic; cook for 2–3 minutes, stirring frequently.

5. Add rice and peas and stir as all ingredients are heated.

6. Reduce heat to medium and stir in tofu and soy sauce mixture; continue to stir until all ingredients are well heated and liquid is absorbed. Serve hot.

Makes 4 servings

Sweet Brown Rice with Spicy Sauce

Steamed short-grain brown rice is almost always available in my home. I love the flavor and the texture. Plus it's so healthy for our bodies. The spicy sauce in this recipe is easy to make and turns simple brown rice into a great showpiece for your meal. Serve it with stir-fried vegetables and a simple salad or fresh fruit and you have a beautiful meal.

INGREDIENTS

- 1 teaspoon olive oil
- 1 yellow onion, chopped
- 3 cloves garlic, minced
- 2 tablespoons minced fresh gingerroot
- ⅓ cup water
- ¼ cup ponzu* (a Japanese sauce found in the Asian foods section of supermarkets)
- ½ teaspoon chili-garlic sauce
- 2 teaspoons sesame oil (also in the Asian foods section)
- 4 tablespoons chopped fresh cilantro, divided
- 4 cups cooked short-grain sweet brown rice

1. Heat olive oil in large skillet over medium-high heat; add onion, garlic, and gingerroot and sauté for about 2 minutes, or until onion softens.

2. Add water, ponzu sauce, chili-garlic sauce, sesame oil, and half of the cilantro; stir until well blended and then reduce heat to medium.

3. Add brown rice and cover pan; continue to cook until rice absorbs most of the liquid and all ingredients are well heated, 5 to 7 minutes.

4. Transfer to serving bowl or individual plates; sprinkle with remaining cilantro to garnish.

Makes 4 servings

*Ponzu is sometimes called Japanese soy sauce but the flavor is very distinct since one of the primary ingredients is yuzu, a Japanese citrus fruit. If you are not able to find ponzu, you can substitute lime juice, although the flavor is very different.

Barley and Black Bean Casserole

Barley is rich in flavor and vitamins. When coupled with beans, you create a complete protein and an excellent meat replacement.

INGREDIENTS

- 1 cup pearl barley, uncooked
- 1¼ cups vegetable broth
- 1¼ cups water
- Cooking spray (olive oil)
- 2 cups sliced fresh mushroom
- 1 cup chopped onion
- ½ cup diced green pepper
- 1 can (15 ounces) black beans, rinsed and drained
- Salt and pepper to taste
- 3 tablespoons sunflower seeds

1. Preheat the oven to 350 degrees.

2. Spread barley on baking sheet; bake at 350 degrees for about 8 minutes until lightly brown. Remove for next step, but keep oven on.

3. Combine barley, broth, and water in a saucepan; bring to boil. Cover, reduce heat, and simmer until barley is tender and liquid is absorbed, about 20 minutes.

4. Coat a nonstick skillet with cooking spray; heat over medium heat, then add mushroom, onion, and green pepper. Sauté until tender.

5. Add barley and beans; season with salt and pepper to taste.

6. Coat a 1½-quart baking dish with cooking spray. Spoon barley and bean mixture into dish. Cover with foil and bake at 350 degrees for 30 minutes or until heated thoroughly.

7. Sprinkle with sunflower seeds and bake uncovered for another 5 minutes.

8. Serve.

Makes 4 servings

Barley Vegetable Bowl

The vegetables in this recipe provide lots of flavor, and the bean and barley combination creates a complete protein. This could become a favorite meal. Add a salad and you have a sure winner.

INGREDIENTS

- 3 tablespoons sunflower oil
- 1 red onion, sliced
- ½ fennel bulb, sliced
- 2 medium carrots, peeled, cut in sticks
- 1 parsnip, sliced
- 1 cup pearl barley
- 4 cups vegetable broth
- 1 teaspoon dried thyme
- ⅔ cup green beans, sliced
- 1 can (15 ounces) pinto beans, drained
- 2 teaspoons chopped parsley

1. Heat the oil over medium heat; gently sauté onion, fennel, carrots, and parsnip for about 10 minutes.
2. Stir in the barley and broth. Bring to a boil; add thyme; cover and gently simmer for 40 minutes.
3. Stir in the green beans and drained pinto beans; continue cooking covered, for 20 more minutes.
4. Ladle barley into serving bowls and sprinkle with chopped parsley before serving.

Makes 6 servings

Whole Wheat Orzo with Tomatoes, Peppers, and Asparagus

Orzo looks a lot like rice, but it's actually pasta. The Rice Select brand of whole wheat orzo is a perfect choice for the Daniel Fast, and the addition of fresh vegetables makes for a pleasant and filling main course. Serve this dish with a green salad and sliced fruit and you have a pleasing meal.

INGREDIENTS

- 1 cup uncooked whole wheat orzo
- 4 tablespoons olive oil, divided

- ½ cup red bell pepper, thinly sliced
- ½ cup yellow bell pepper, thinly sliced
- ½ cup green bell pepper, thinly sliced
- 2 tablespoons garlic, minced
- 1 pound asparagus, trimmed and cut into 1½-inch pieces
- ¼ cup fresh basil, minced
- ¼ cup fresh Italian parsley, minced
- ¼ cup fresh mint, minced
- 1 cup diced fresh tomato

1. Cook orzo according to package directions; rinse, drain, and transfer to bowl; toss with 2 tablespoons olive oil.

2. Heat 2 tablespoons olive oil in a large frying pan over medium-high heat. Add red, yellow, and green peppers, along with asparagus and garlic. Sauté until softened.

3. Add basil, parsley, mint, diced tomato, and cooked orzo to frying pan. Gently blend until well heated. Add a little more olive oil if necessary.

4. Transfer to a large bowl and serve hot.

Makes 8 servings

Red Sauce for Whole Wheat Pasta

This is a very basic recipe for red sauce that you can use with whole wheat pasta. Use this recipe as is, or be creative and add ingredients that you enjoy, such as black or kalamata olives, capers, or mushrooms.

INGREDIENTS

- 2 tablespoons olive oil
- 1 green bell pepper, diced large
- 1 yellow onion, diced large
- 2 cloves garlic, minced
- 2 cans (15 ounces each) diced tomatoes
- 2 cans (15 ounces each) tomato sauce
- 1 tablespoon Italian herbs
- Salt and freshly ground black pepper to taste

1. Heat the oil in a large skillet over medium-high heat. Add the bell pepper, onion, and garlic; sauté until the bell pepper softens, 5 to 7 minutes.

2. Add the tomatoes, tomato sauce, and Italian herbs. Reduce heat to medium-low and allow to simmer for 30 minutes. Season to taste with the salt and pepper.

3. Serve over hot pasta of your choice.

Makes 6 servings

Salads

It's likely that you will eat more salads than usual while on the Daniel Fast. Your body will be happy, and so will your waistline! Salads are a superb way to consume the fiber your body needs along with the flavors and textures your mouth desires.

Most of the recipes in this section can be used for side salads. Plus many can serve as a main course. As you create your salads, consider asking family members to help. This is a great way to get children to eat salads.

A great time-saving tip is to wash and prepare all the salad ingredients at one time. It's great to open the fridge, grab three handfuls of mixed greens, ½ cup of sliced scallions, 1 cup of diced red pepper, add a premade dressing, and create a great salad with virtually no work at all. To really win points with the family, offer a wide variety of additional ingredients in small bowls (sunflower seeds, black beans, capers, and red onion slices for starters) so everyone can dress up their salads to their liking.

Garnish Ideas:
- Beans (kidney, pinto, or black beans, chickpeas, etc.), drained and rinsed
- Seeds (sunflower, pumpkin, poppy)
- Nuts (slivered almonds, walnuts, pecans, peanuts, cashews, etc.)
- Fresh fruit (strawberries, oranges, grapefruit, grapes, pomegranate, etc.)
- Dried fruit (raisins, apricots, dates, prunes)
- Coconut
- Onions
- Olives
- Capers
- Beets
- Green peas or pea pods
- Cucumber slices
- Mushrooms

White Bean Salad with Tomatoes and Herbs

I not only love the flavors of this recipe, but the colors are also appetizing. The contrast between the white beans, the red tomatoes, and the green lettuce, onions, and herbs is lovely!

INGREDIENTS

- 2 cans (15 ounces each) navy or cannellini beans, rinsed and drained
- 2 cups seeded and diced tomato
- ½ cup chopped celery
- ⅓ cup shredded carrot
- ⅓ cup chopped scallions
- ¼ cup chopped fresh parsley
- 1 tablespoon minced shallots
- ¼ cup white wine vinegar
- 2 tablespoons extra-virgin olive oil
- 2 teaspoons Dijon mustard
- 1 teaspoon minced fresh rosemary
- 1 teaspoon minced fresh thyme
- Salt (optional)
- Freshly ground black pepper
- 4 cups shredded green leaf lettuce

1. In a large bowl, toss together the beans, tomato, celery, carrot, scallions, parsley, and shallots.

2. In a small bowl, whisk together the vinegar, oil, mustard, rosemary, thyme, salt (if using), and pepper to taste.

3. Pour over the salad mixture and toss gently. Serve on a bed of lettuce on individual salad plates.

Makes 4 servings

Asian Noodle Salad

You'll be coming back for more on this recipe. The great flavor of the whole wheat noodles adds a richness to these typical Asian flavors that makes this salad recipe a real keeper.

INGREDIENTS

- 8 ounces whole wheat thin spaghetti noodles
- 2 tablespoons canola oil
- ¼ cup chopped fresh cilantro

- 3 tablespoons soy sauce
- 2 tablespoons fresh lemon or lime juice
- 1 tablespoon minced garlic
- 1 teaspoon minced fresh ginger
- 1 teaspoon sesame oil
- 1 teaspoon creamy peanut butter
- ⅛ teaspoon red pepper flakes
- 1 cup peeled, seeded, and sliced cucumber
- 1 cup sliced snow peas
- ½ cup diced red bell pepper
- ½ cup pineapple chunks, cut in half
- ⅛ teaspoon salt
- ⅛ teaspoon ground black pepper

1. Bring a large pot of water to a boil. Cook the noodles according to package directions until al dente. Drain well (do not rinse), toss with canola oil, and set aside.

2. In a large bowl, combine the cilantro, soy sauce, lemon juice, garlic, ginger, oil, peanut butter, and red pepper flakes. Stir until well blended.

3. Add the cucumber, snow peas, bell pepper, pineapple chunks, and noodles, and toss. Let stand, covered, at room temperature for 1 hour, stirring occasionally so the flavors soak into the vegetables and pineapple.

4. Adjust the seasoning with the salt and pepper, toss again, and serve.

Makes 4 servings

Roasted Asparagus with Tomato Basil Vinaigrette

I have the great joy of having wild asparagus growing near my home. So I especially like this recipe that adorns the spears with color and flavor!

INGREDIENTS

- 2 pounds thin asparagus spears, trimmed
- 1 tablespoon olive oil
- Salt and freshly ground black pepper
- 1 medium tomato, cored, seeded, and minced
- 1 medium shallot, minced
- 1½ tablespoons lemon juice
- 1 tablespoon minced fresh basil leaves
- 3 tablespoons extra-virgin olive oil

1. If using an electric stove, place oven rack to uppermost position and then heat the broiler.

2. Toss the trimmed asparagus with oil and then season with salt and pepper; lay asparagus spears in single layer on heavy-rimmed baking sheet (I like to line it with foil for easy cleanup).

3. Place baking sheet on top oven rack or use the broiler in a gas stove and broil about 4 inches from heating element, shaking pan halfway through to turn spears; broil until asparagus is tender and lightly browned, 8 to 10 minutes.

4. Allow spears to cool, and then arrange on serving dish.

5. Whisk tomato, shallot, lemon juice, basil, and olive oil in a small bowl; season to taste with salt and pepper and then drizzle over asparagus; serve at room temperature.

Makes 6–8 servings

Bean and Pasta Salad

This bean and pasta salad is so versatile. It can serve as a lunch entrée or a side dish for dinner. The salad packs well for lunches, so consider this recipe as a great option for work or school.

INGREDIENTS

- 1½ cups cooked or canned pink or red beans
- 2 cups small shell pasta, cooked, drained, and tossed with a small amount of olive oil
- 2 cups frozen peas and carrots, thawed and drained
- ½ cup sliced celery

Dressing

- ¼ cup prepared seasoned oil and vinegar dressing (consider Newman's Own Oil and Vinegar Salad Dressing)
- ¼ cup soynnaise
- 2 tablespoons chopped Italian parsley
- ½ teaspoon salt
- ⅛ teaspoon freshly ground black pepper

1. Combine beans, pasta, peas and carrots, and celery. Add the prepared salad dressing, soynnaise, parsley, salt, and pepper and toss until blended.

2. If desired, refrigerate for at least 1 hour before serving; or serve at room temperature.

Makes 8 servings

Just a Little Oil Does the Trick
Tossing cooked and drained pasta with a little oil will keep the noodles, macaroni, or other pasta shapes from sticking together.

Cabbage, Apple, and Ginger Salad

This tasty salad is full of interesting flavors as the ginger, celery seed, and sweet apple hit your palate. It's quick to make and a good keeper, so make it ahead and pull it from the fridge when mealtime comes around.

INGREDIENTS

- 2 tablespoons rice vinegar
- ¼ cup lime juice
- 1 teaspoon grated, peeled fresh ginger
- ¼ cup walnut or vegetable oil
- ½ teaspoon celery seed
- ¼ teaspoon salt
- ⅛ teaspoon freshly ground black pepper
- 4 cups (about ¼ head) shredded green cabbage
- 2 large sweet apples, unpeeled and cut into matchsticks

1. Whisk the vinegar, lime juice, and ginger in a large mixing bowl. Gradually add the oil and whisk with each addition; add celery seed, salt, and pepper.

2. Add the cabbage and apples and gently toss to coat.

3. Refrigerate for 30 minutes before serving.

Makes 6 servings

Curried Bean and Rice Salad

Here's a flavorful and nutritious salad that works well for a meal. The colors are inviting, and the curry offers mouth-satisfying goodness.

INGREDIENTS

- 1 tablespoon canola oil
- 1 teaspoon curry powder

- ¾ cup vegetable broth
- ⅓ cup uncooked long-grain brown rice
- ¼ cup chopped celery
- 2 tablespoons chopped scallion
- 2 tablespoons chopped green bell pepper
- 1 tablespoon lime juice
- 2 cups cooked and drained light or dark red kidney beans (you can also substitute with canned beans)
- ¼ cup soynnaise
- 2 tablespoons toasted slivered almonds
- ¼ teaspoon salt
- Freshly ground black pepper
- 1 tomato, cut into wedges
- Parsley sprigs

1. Heat oil in large saucepan over medium heat; add curry powder and sauté several seconds, then stir in vegetable broth; increase heat to bring to a boil.

2. Add rice; cover and adjust heat to simmer for 20 minutes or until all liquid is absorbed and rice is cooked.

3. Stir in celery, scallion, green pepper, and lime juice. Chill thoroughly in refrigerator for 1 to 2 hours.

4. Just before serving, add beans, soynnaise, and almonds into rice mixture. Adjust seasoning with salt and pepper.

5. Garnish with tomato and parsley and serve.

Makes 4 servings

Fennel, Olive, and Orange Salad

This scrumptious salad is a colorful blend of flavors that serves as a refreshing side dish for spicy entrées. Serve on separate plates or in a salad bowl for a lovely presentation.

INGREDIENTS

- 3 fennel bulbs, tops removed
- 1 tablespoon fresh lemon juice
- 1 pound mixed green salad mix
- 2 oranges, peeled and sectioned with membranes removed

- ⅓ cup pitted kalamata or Greek green olives, halved lengthwise
- ½ cup fresh Italian parsley leaves
- ¼ cup fresh orange juice
- ¼ cup extra-virgin olive oil
- 1 teaspoon salt
- ¼ teaspoon freshly ground black pepper

1. Cut each fennel bulb in half, then thinly slice.
2. Place sliced fennel into salad bowl and toss with fresh lemon juice.
3. Add salad greens, oranges, olives, and parsley and gently toss until well blended.
4. In a small bowl, whisk the orange juice and olive oil together until emulsified. Season with salt and pepper and whisk again.
5. Just before serving, pour the dressing over salad mixture and toss.

Makes 8 servings

Fresh Corn Salad

This recipe is best when fresh corn is available. The colors are great, and the flavors mouthwatering. It's a favorite for all, and a wonderful addition to your meal.

INGREDIENTS

- 8 ears corn, shucked and ready to boil
- ¾ cup finely diced red onion
- 5 tablespoons cider vinegar
- 5 tablespoons olive oil
- ¾ teaspoon kosher salt
- Freshly ground black pepper to taste
- ¾ cup fresh basil leaves, thinly sliced

1. Fill a large pot with water, add salt, and bring to boil; carefully place ears of corn in water and cook for 3 minutes, or until starchiness is just gone.
2. Drain corn and immerse in ice water to stop cooking; when cool, cut kernels off cob, cutting close to but avoiding the cob.
3. Place the corn in a large bowl; add red onion, vinegar, olive oil, kosher salt, and freshly ground black pepper to your liking.

4. Just before serving, add the fresh basil and toss; adjust seasoning to taste. Serve cold or at room temperature.

Makes 8 servings

Yikes! Corn Is All Over My Kitchen

To avoid this mishap, cut the cobs in a bowl in your sink. Cleanup will be much easier!

Garden Fresh Bean Salad

This is another unique bean salad that can be served as a side dish or a flavorful lunch entrée.

INGREDIENTS

- 2 cans (15 ounces each) kidney beans, rinsed and drained
- 2 cans (15 ounces each) chickpeas, rinsed and drained
- 2 carrots, grated
- 1 small zucchini, diced
- 5 radishes, sliced
- ⅔ cup olive or vegetable oil
- ⅓ cup cider or red wine vinegar
- 1 teaspoon Italian seasoning
- ½ teaspoon salt
- ½ teaspoon garlic powder
- ½ teaspoon onion powder
- 8–10 green lettuce leaves

1. Using a large bowl, combine the kidney beans, chickpeas, carrots, zucchini, and radishes.

2. In a smaller bowl, combine the oil, vinegar, Italian seasoning, salt, garlic powder, and onion powder. Pour this dressing over vegetable mixture and toss to coat.

3. Cover and refrigerate the salad for at least 2 hours.

4. With a slotted spoon, dish up servings of salad onto plates lined with lettuce leaves.

Makes 8–10 servings

Daniel Fast Greek Salad

Okay, I want to warn you that a Greek salad without feta cheese is slightly lacking. But after all, we are on a fast where we restrict some foods. This recipe is a great way to enjoy a Greek salad, even though you might miss that one ingredient. The good news is that this salad is still packed with color, nutrition, and flavor so it's good to look at, good for you, and pleasant to your taste buds!

Vinaigrette

- 3 tablespoons red wine vinegar
- 1½ teaspoons lemon juice from 1 lemon
- 2 teaspoons minced fresh oregano leaves
- ½ teaspoon table salt
- ⅛ teaspoon ground black pepper
- 1 clove garlic, minced
- 6 tablespoons olive oil

1. Whisk vinaigrette ingredients in large bowl until combined. This can be prepared earlier in the day and set aside until you are ready to prepare the salad. Otherwise, proceed to salad recipe.

Salad

- ½ red onion, thinly sliced (about ¾ cup)
- 1 cucumber, peeled, halved lengthwise, seeded, and cut into ⅛-inch-thick slices
- 2 hearts romaine lettuce, washed, dried thoroughly, and torn into bite-sized pieces
- 2 large vine-ripened tomatoes, cored, seeded, and cut into 12 wedges
- ¼ cup loosely packed torn fresh Italian parsley leaves
- ¼ cup loosely packed torn fresh mint leaves
- 1 jar (6 ounces) roasted red bell pepper, cut into long bite-size strips
- 20 large pitted kalamata olives, quartered lengthwise

1. Add onion and cucumber to the bowl with the prepared vinaigrette dressing and toss; let stand to blend flavors (about 20 minutes).

2. Add the romaine lettuce, tomato wedges, parsley, mint, and peppers to the bowl with the onions and cucumber in the prepared vinaigrette dressing; gently toss to coat with dressing.

3. Serve in one large bowl or platter or arrange on individual serving plates; sprinkle olives over salad and serve.

Makes 6–8 servings

Green Salad with Walnut Dressing

This vitamin-packed dressing is so good and will keep for several days in an air-tight container in the fridge. Walnut oil has a nutty aroma and a delicate nutty flavor. It should only be used on cold foods, as heating the oil can cause it to lose its flavor and turn bitter. Walnut oil is more expensive, but I find it well worth the extra cost for the flavor. However, there are times when I make this same recipe with extra-virgin olive oil, and it's still very enjoyable.

INGREDIENTS

- 2 cups baby spinach leaves
- ½ cup lightly packed parsley leaves
- ⅓ cup lightly packed fresh dill
- ¼ cup walnut or olive oil
- 2 tablespoons vegetable broth
- 4 teaspoons apple cider vinegar
- ¼ teaspoon salt
- ⅛ teaspoon ground black pepper
- 8 cups mixed salad greens, torn in bite-sized pieces
- ¼ cup walnuts, chopped for garnish

1. Place the spinach, parsley, dill, oil, broth, vinegar, salt, and pepper in a blender or food processor. Process until the dressing is smooth and slightly thickened (you may need to scrape the sides once or twice while processing).

2. Place the mixed salad greens in a large bowl and drizzle the dressing over the top and toss. Use this bowl to serve or transfer to individual serving dishes. Sprinkle with chopped walnuts and serve.

Makes 4 servings

Add Some Color!

I also use this salad as a "canvas" of sorts and then add sliced fruit to sweeten it up. Consider strawberries, grapes, oranges, or pineapple. You can also use pecans or slivered almonds as substitutes for the walnuts.

Susan's Favorite Cucumber, Bell Pepper, and Tomato Salad

This is one of my favorite recipes because it's so easy and so refreshing. I love the colors and texture of the salad, and the dressing is a real winner too!

INGREDIENTS

- 1 English cucumber, cut in half lengthwise, remove seeds, cut into ½-inch slices
- 1 red bell pepper, cored, diced large
- 1 yellow bell pepper, cored, diced large
- 1 pint cherry tomatoes, cut in half lengthwise
- 1 small red onion, diced large
- ½ cup kalamata olives

Salad Dressing

- ½ cup extra-virgin olive oil
- ¼ cup red wine vinegar
- 1 teaspoon dried oregano (rub between hands to release oils)
- 2 cloves garlic, minced
- ½ teaspoon Dijon mustard
- 1 teaspoon salt
- ½ teaspoon pepper

1. Emulsify all the salad dressing ingredients together in a small bowl; set aside.

2. Using a large bowl, gently toss the cucumber, red and yellow bell peppers, tomatoes, red onion, and olives together.

3. Whisk the dressing again before pouring it over the salad; toss again and serve.

Makes 6 servings

Mediterranean Tofu Salad

This is one of my favorite salads to enjoy for lunch or dinner. The tofu adds more than 10 grams of protein per serving, and absorbs the flavorful dressing.

INGREDIENTS

- 2 tablespoons extra-virgin olive oil
- 1 tablespoon balsamic vinegar

- 1 teaspoon Dijon mustard
- ½ teaspoon dried chives (or 1 teaspoon fresh chives)
- Salt and pepper to taste
- 1 package (16 ounces) firm tofu, drained, blotted dry, cut into ¾-inch cubes
- 4 cups mixed salad greens, torn into bite-sized pieces
- 4 marinated sun-dried tomatoes, drained and chopped
- ¼ cup chopped nuts (such as pecans, walnuts, slivered almonds)

1. Whisk together in a small bowl the oil, vinegar, mustard, and chives, and then add salt and pepper to taste.

2. Place the diced tofu in a separate bowl and gently toss with about 1 tablespoon of dressing, making sure each piece is well coated.

3. Place the mixed salad greens in a large bowl and toss with the remaining dressing. Arrange greens on four plates and scatter tofu and tomatoes over each serving. Top with chopped nuts if desired.

Makes 4 servings

Sweet Potato Salad

This is a wonderful alternative to the classic potato salad, and it has more nutrition and fewer calories. To top those benefits, this salad is packed with flavor and it looks good. This recipe is a winner in my house!

INGREDIENTS

- 4 orange-fleshed yams (or sweet potatoes)
- ¼ cup soynnaise
- 1 tablespoon Dijon mustard
- 4 ribs celery, cut into ¼-inch slices
- 1 small red bell pepper, seeded and cut in small dices
- 1 cup diced fresh pineapple
- 2 scallions, white and green parts, finely chopped
- Salt and freshly ground black pepper
- ½ cup coarsely chopped pecans, toasted
- ¼ cup roughly chopped fresh chives, for garnish

1. Preheat the oven to 400 degrees.

2. Wrap the individual potatoes in foil and bake for 1 hour or until tender.

3. Cool the potatoes until they are easy to handle. Peel and then cut into ¾-inch chunks.

4. In a large bowl, mix the soynnaise and mustard. Add the yams, celery, red pepper, pineapple, and scallions and toss gently, seasoning to taste with salt and pepper.

5. Cover and refrigerate for at least 1 hour. This salad can be made one day ahead, covered, and refrigerated. Be sure to adjust the seasonings before serving.

6. Just before serving, fold in the pecans and garnish with the chives. Serve chilled.

Makes 8 servings

Yams or Sweet Potatoes?
While they seem to be similar, technically the yam and sweet potato are not even closely related! The sweet potato is the tuber of a morning glory vine, and the yam (which is sweeter) is the tuber of a tropical vine. Yams are becoming more commonly used in the United States. While these two foods don't show up close to each other on botanical charts, they can usually be interchanged in recipes.

Full Meal Green Salad

My friends Scott and Anna Andrews invited me to their home for dinner while I was on the Daniel Fast. In Anna's always loving way, she prepared a wonderful meal that suited everyone, even though I was the only one fasting. This salad was the main course, and the Spicy Three Bean Salad that follows was a side dish. It was so appetizing, flavorful, and filling that I asked Anna if I could share the recipes with you!

INGREDIENTS
- 3 cups bok choy, leaves and stalks
- 2 cups romaine
- 1 cup red cabbage, coarsely chopped
- 2 cups zucchini, coarsely chopped
- 3 scallions, diced
- ½ cup fresh green beans, cut in ½-inch pieces
- ¾ cup cherry tomatoes, halved

Garnishes
- 1 can (15 ounces) black beans, rinsed and drained
- 1 cup black olives
- 1 cup pine nuts or sunflower seeds

1. Using a large salad bowl, prepare bok choy leaves and romaine as for any salad, cutting the bok choy stalk into ½-inch chunks. Add cabbage, zucchini, scallions, green beans, and tomatoes; gently toss.

2. Place the following ingredients in individual small serving bowls: black beans, black olives, and pine nuts/sunflower seeds so diners can garnish their own salads.

3. Serve with your favorite Daniel Fast–friendly dressings (refer to Salad Dressings on page 195).

Makes 6 servings

Spicy Three Bean Salad

This is my friend Anna Andrews's recipe, and it's so good! The spiciness in the pickled vegetables is a great contrast for a lettuce salad (see above).

INGREDIENTS

- 1 jar spicy dilly beans (pickled green beans) or asparagus
- 1 jar (7 ounces) spicy pickled carrots/cauliflower
- 1 can (15 ounces) kidney beans, rinsed
- 1 can (15 ounces) chickpeas, rinsed
- ¼ cup diced red onion

1. Cut dilly beans (or asparagus) into ½-inch sections and combine with carrots/cauliflower, juices included. Add in kidney beans, chickpeas, and diced onion; gently toss.

2. Serve in a medium-sized bowl with a slotted spoon.

Makes 6 servings

Black Bean and Mango Salad

You and everyone you serve this salad to will be wanting more of this yummy dish. The sweetness of the fresh mango and the flavors of the beans and red bell peppers will give your taste buds a joyful workout! Plus each serving is packed with protein, fiber, and nutrients. This is a great salad to make ahead.

INGREDIENTS

- 1 ripe mango, peeled, pitted, diced, divided
- 6 tablespoons olive oil
- 2 tablespoons white wine vinegar
- 2 tablespoons chopped fresh parsley

- 1 tablespoon fresh lemon juice
- 2 garlic cloves, chopped
- 1 teaspoon dried basil, crumbled
- ¼ teaspoon dried crushed red pepper flakes
- Pinch of dried oregano
- 2 cans (15 ounces each) black beans, drained and rinsed
- 1 can (15 ounces) chickpeas, drained and rinsed
- ½ cup chopped red onion
- 1 red bell pepper, chopped
- Salt and pepper to taste

1. Measure ⅓ cup of the diced mango and place it in a blender; add the olive oil, vinegar, parsley, lemon juice, garlic cloves, basil, red pepper flakes, and oregano. Blend until smooth, about 1 minute.

2. In a large bowl, add the remainder of the diced mango, black beans, chickpeas, red onion, and red bell pepper. Pour the mango dressing over the mixture and gently toss. Adjust seasoning with salt and pepper.

3. For best results, chill the salad for at least 1 hour before serving.

Makes 4 servings

Tangy Bean and Spinach Salad

Serve this salad as a main course or as a side dish. Either way, it's an enjoyable dish with lots of color, texture, flavor, and nutrients.

INGREDIENTS

- 1 can (15 ounces) pinto beans or lima beans or 1½ cups cooked dry-packaged pinto beans or lima beans, rinsed and drained
- 1 cup cauliflower florets
- 1 cup chopped red bell pepper
- 1 small avocado, peeled, pitted, cubed
- 2 scallions with tops, sliced
- ½ cup prepared oil and vinegar dressing (consider using Newman's Own Oil and Vinegar Salad Dressing)
- 4 cups baby spinach leaves
- 1 can (11 ounces) mandarin orange segments, drained, or 1 fresh orange, peeled, chopped
- 2 tablespoons toasted sunflower seeds, optional

1. Combine the beans, cauliflower, bell pepper, avocado, and scallions in a salad bowl by tossing gently.

2. Pour the dressing over the salad and gently toss again.

3. Add spinach and oranges and lightly toss.

4. Sprinkle with sunflower seeds before serving in a serving bowl or on individual salad plates.

Makes 4 entrée servings or 8 side dish servings

Tomato Salad with Walnuts

Tomatoes and walnuts isn't a common combination, but it sure is pleasant! This is a quick and easy salad to put together and is a great accompaniment for soup, chili, or some other hearty main dish.

INGREDIENTS

- ¼ cup walnut oil
- 1½ tablespoons lemon juice
- 1 small garlic clove, minced
- 2 teaspoons chopped fresh tarragon
- ⅛ teaspoon salt
- ⅛ teaspoon freshly ground black pepper
- 4 tomatoes, sliced
- 1 red onion, sliced
- 2 tablespoons chopped walnuts

1. Whisk the oil, lemon juice, garlic, tarragon, salt, and pepper in a small bowl. You might want to make the dressing ahead; it stores well in a covered container in the refrigerator for up to 3 days.

2. Using a serving platter or individual plates, overlap the tomato and onion slices in an alternating pattern until all the slices have been used.

3. Drizzle with the tarragon-garlic mixture and then sprinkle with the chopped walnuts.

Makes 4 servings

Always Ready Fresh Green Salad

I love those cello bags of prepared salad greens for quick meals. But truthfully, they are expensive and in my experience seem to spoil sooner than when I purchase heads of lettuce. So I try to make my own blends of greens by purchasing a few heads of different varieties of lettuce. At home, I wash, tear, and spin the greens and then store them in a large airtight container. I place a couple of layers of paper towel on top of the greens to absorb any evaporating liquid. This seems to keep the greens fresh longer. I also prepare several days of "salad fixins" at one time and keep the individual ingredients in the fridge. When I need a salad, I can just grab a couple of handfuls of the prepared greens, add a few other vegetables along with a simple homemade salad dressing, and "Presto!" Salad's ready!

INGREDIENTS

- 1 head green leaf lettuce
- 1 head red leaf lettuce
- 1 head Bibb or other type of lettuce
- 1 bunch scallions, trimmed and sliced
- 1 bunch radishes, trimmed and sliced
- 1 English cucumber, sliced as needed
- 1 carrot, coarsely grated or thinly sliced
- 1 red bell pepper, sliced or slivered
- 1 red onion, halved and then cut into half rings
- 1 can (11 ounces) mandarin oranges
- 1 cup almonds, slivered or sliced

1. Wash and tear all the lettuce greens; spin them in salad spinner, removing as much water as possible. Store greens in large airtight container, placing two layers of paper towel atop the greens to absorb moisture before sealing.

2. Trim and cut all other salad vegetables and store in airtight containers until ready to use.

3. During the week, use prepared greens and then add two or three other ingredients to make creative and tasty salads quickly. Add your favorite homemade dressing just before serving.

4. Be sure to use all ingredients throughout the week to avoid waste.

Makes 8–10 servings

Avocado, Orange, Olive, and Almond Spanish Salad

Making salads that are rich in flavor, color, and texture make them more appetizing and satisfying. This salad is an excellent choice for an interesting mix of sweet and salty. Be sure to use a flavorful olive, such as the kalamata variety, as they add the special zip that really suits this recipe.

INGREDIENTS

Dressing

- 4 tablespoons extra-virgin olive oil
- 2 tablespoons freshly squeezed lemon juice
- 1 tablespoon finely chopped Italian parsley

Salad

- 2 avocados, peeled, seeded, and cut into chunks
- 2 tomatoes, peeled, seeded, and cut into bite-size pieces
- Salt and pepper to taste
- 2 naval oranges, peeled and sliced into thick rounds
- 1 small white onion, sliced into rings
- ¼ cup sliced almonds
- 1 cup pitted kalamata olives

1. Using a small bowl, whisk together the olive oil, lemon juice, and parsley until well blended.

2. Place the avocado chunks in a separate bowl and toss with half the dressing so that all pieces are well covered. This will retain the fresh color of the avocados; add the tomatoes and then season with salt and pepper; gently toss.

3. Arrange the orange slices on a large round or oval serving plate, then spread the onion rings over the oranges.

4. Spoon the avocados and tomatoes in the center of the plate. Sprinkle with almond slices and garnish with olives.

5. Whisk the remaining dressing and pour over the salad just before serving.

Makes 4 servings

Red, Black, and Yellow Delight Salad

Have you ever made a recipe that is so good that you just have to keep sampling it before serving it to your family? Well, this is one of those gems. You might want to double this delightful recipe to make sure there's enough for a couple of meals . . . and for your taste tests!

INGREDIENTS

- 1 can (15 ounces) black beans, rinsed and drained
- 2 cups frozen corn kernels
- 1 small red bell pepper, seeded and chopped
- ½ red onion, chopped
- 2 stalks celery, cut into small dices
- 1½ teaspoons ground cumin
- 1–2 teaspoons hot sauce (I recommend Tabasco brand)
- 1 lime, juiced
- 2 tablespoons vegetable or olive oil
- Salt and pepper
- 4 lettuce leaves to use for serving (optional)

1. Place all the ingredients (except the lettuce leaves) in a large bowl and then lightly toss.

2. Allow the salad to stand at room temperature for at least 15 minutes, which allows the flavors to fuse, and gives time for the corn to thaw while keeping all the other ingredients chilled.

3. Gently stir the salad before spooning it onto the lettuce-lined plates.

Makes 4 servings

Persian Salad

This simple salad is quick to prepare and a pleasant addition to your Daniel Fast lunch or dinner menu. Consider preparing the tomatoes, cucumber, and onion in advance so when mealtime arrives you can make this salad in just a few minutes.

INGREDIENTS

- 4 tomatoes, seeded and diced into small cubes
- ½ cucumber, peeled, seeded, and diced into small cubes
- 1 white onion, finely chopped
- 1 head green leaf lettuce, torn into bite-size pieces

Dressing

- 2 tablespoons olive oil
- 1 lemon, juiced
- 1 clove garlic, crushed and finely minced
- Salt and pepper to taste

1. Place the tomatoes, cucumber, onion, and lettuce in a serving bowl and gently toss to mix them together.
2. Using a small bowl, whisk together the olive oil, lemon juice, and garlic. Whisk together until emulsified, and then season with salt and pepper to taste.
3. Just before serving, pour the dressing over the salad and toss lightly to mix. Sprinkle with more freshly ground black pepper.

Makes 4 servings

Turkish Salad

This salad is a delicious combination of flavors, textures, and colors. The tasty salad vegetables are even more flavorful with the herb dressing.

INGREDIENTS

- 1 head green leaf lettuce, torn into bite-size pieces
- 4 tomatoes, seeded and diced into small cubes
- 1 green bell pepper, cut into thin strips
- 1 red bell pepper, cut into thin strips
- ½ cucumber, peeled, seeded, and sliced
- 1 red onion, cut in half and then sliced into half-rings
- 1 cup pitted black olives (such as kalamata), either sliced or served whole

Dressing

- 3 tablespoons extra-virgin olive oil
- 3 tablespoons freshly squeezed lemon juice
- 1 clove garlic, crushed and finely minced
- 1 tablespoon finely chopped fresh Italian parsley
- 1 tablespoon finely chopped fresh mint
- Salt and pepper to taste

1. Place the lettuce, tomatoes, green pepper, red pepper, cucumber, and onion in salad serving bowl. Gently toss to mix vegetables.

2. In a separate bowl, whisk together the olive oil and lemon juice until emulsified. Add garlic, parsley, and mint, and mix again until blended. Season to taste with salt and pepper.

3. Just before serving, whisk the dressing again, pour over salad vegetables, and toss. Add olives and gently toss again. Serve.

Makes 4 servings

Add 1 Cup Efficiency and Stir

To save meal preparation time, consider doubling or even tripling this salad dressing recipe to use later in the week. Store in an airtight container in the fridge for several days.

Asian Salad

Serve this salad with the Faux Fried Rice (page 167) for a fun and pleasant meal. You can also double the salad dressing recipe to store in the refrigerator for future meals.

INGREDIENTS

- 1 head green leaf lettuce, torn into bite-size pieces
- 1 can (11 ounces) mandarin orange pieces, drained, or 1 orange, peeled and sections cut into bite-size pieces
- 1 can (5 ounces) sliced water chestnuts
- 1 small red onion, sliced and then separated into rings
- ½ cup slivered almonds or ¼ cup toasted sesame seeds

Dressing

- 2 tablespoons extra-virgin olive oil
- 1 tablespoon soy sauce
- 2 tablespoons peanut oil
- 2 teaspoons tomato paste
- 1–2 teaspoons apple juice (from frozen concentrate)
- 2 tablespoons chopped carrot
- 2 tablespoons chopped celery
- 2 tablespoons chopped onion
- 2 teaspoons chopped gingerroot (remove peel before slicing)

1. Place the lettuce, orange pieces, water chestnuts, and onion slices in a bowl; toss.

2. Place all dressing ingredients in a blender and liquefy until smooth.

3. Adjust seasoning with soy sauce or salt; adjust sweetness with apple juice.

4. Just before serving, whisk the salad dressing and then toss with salad vegetables, adding just enough dressing to cover.

5. Garnish the salad with almonds or sesame seeds and serve.

Makes 4 servings

New Chopped Vegetable Salad with Vinaigrette

This salad is fashioned after one prepared by Wolfgang Puck and served at Chinois, his famous restaurant in Santa Monica, California. This adaptation has lots of color and flavor, and is Daniel Fast friendly! Serve with a simple hot soup for a complete meal.

INGREDIENTS

- ½ cup diced green beans
- ½ cup diced red onion
- ½ cup diced Belgian endive
- ½ cup diced artichoke hearts
- ½ cup fresh or frozen corn kernels
- ½ cup diced celery
- ½ cup diced radishes
- ½ cup diced avocado
- ¼ cup chopped tomato, peeled and seeded first
- 1 cup mixed salad greens of your choice, cut or torn into bite-sized pieces

Vinaigrette

- 1 tablespoon Dijon mustard
- 3 tablespoons balsamic or red wine vinegar*
- ½ cup extra-virgin olive oil
- ½ cup canola oil
- Salt and freshly ground black pepper to taste

1. Place the beans in a sieve; then set the sieve into boiling water so vegetables will blanch; cook for 2 to 3 minutes. Lift the sieve from the boiling water and place in ice water to stop cooking; drain.

2. Place the cooled beans in a large salad bowl; add red onion, endive, artichoke hearts, corn kernels, celery, and radishes; toss to combine.

3. Just before serving, prepare and add the avocado and tomato.

4. Prepare the vinaigrette by combining the mustard and vinegar in a small bowl. Slowly whisk in the oils to emulsify the mixture. Season to taste with salt and pepper. (You can make the dressing ahead of time; just whisk before using.)

5. Divide dressing into two equal portions; dress the mixed vegetables with some or all of one portion; in a separate bowl, dress the lettuce with some or all of the second portion.

6. To serve, divide the lettuce onto four individual salad plates; add mounds of the vegetable mixture to the top of the lettuce, dividing portions equally.

7. Salt and pepper to taste.

Makes 4 servings

*Wine vinegars are not alcoholic and, therefore, are allowed on the Daniel Fast, whereas drinking any alcohol is not allowed.

New Daniel Fast Caesar Salad

While this is slightly different from the traditional Caesar salad, it's a great option for the Daniel Fast. Instead of eggs, pulverized almonds and tofu create the creamy texture of the dressing. For best results, make the dressing at least an hour ahead so the flavors have time to merge and the dressing is well chilled.

INGREDIENTS

- ½ cup slivered or sliced blanched almonds
- 4 cloves garlic, peeled and crushed
- ¾ pound silken tofu
- ¼ cup olive oil
- 3 tablespoons lemon juice
- 1 tablespoon capers (or 4 Greek green olives, chopped)
- 1 tablespoon plus 1 teaspoon caper brine
- ½ teaspoon mustard powder
- 1 large head romaine lettuce, cut or torn into bite-sized pieces (or cut the head into quarters lengthwise, keeping the core intact; serve each quarter whole with drizzled dressing)
- 3 green onions, chopped (optional)
- Salt and freshly ground pepper to taste

1. Pulse almonds in a food processor or blender until ground (like cornmeal); place in container with airtight lid (all other dressing ingredients will be added to it, so choose size accordingly).

2. Mix garlic, tofu, and oil in the food processor or blender until creamy; add lemon juice, capers or olives, caper brine, and mustard powder. Pulse until just blended.

3. Season with salt and pepper. Add more lemon juice if desired.

4. Pour mixture into container with the ground almonds, and whisk until well blended. Cover and chill between 30 and 90 minutes.

5. Just before serving, toss lettuce and green onions; add dressing in small portions as you toss the salad so each piece of lettuce is just lightly coated.

Makes 4 side servings or 2 main course servings

Salad Dressings

Finding a prepared dressing suitable for the Daniel Fast is nearly impossible. Most have sweetener added and many also have chemicals and dairy products.

The one dressing I've found that is perfect for the fast is Newman's Own Oil and Vinegar Salad Dressing. Still, making your own dressings is a snap and really fast once you learn some simple principles:

1. Your salad dressing should complement the tastes of the salad ingredients.

2. There are two major categories of dressings: vinaigrettes and creamy-style dressings. Vinaigrettes have oil and an acid agent mixed together until they are emulsified (blending two ingredients that normally don't mix together, such as oil and vinegar). Creamy dressings usually include mayonnaise (soynnaise for the Daniel Fast) and are also commonly emulsified.

3. Vinaigrettes usually use a ratio of one part vinegar or acidic juice to three parts oil, varied by added herbs and spices. First mix the liquid with the herbs, spices, and salt, and then slowly drizzle the oil into the mixture while whisking until the dressing is emulsified and thick. Serve immediately, or set aside and whisk again before dressing your salad.

Basic Oil, Vinegar, and Herb Salad Dressing

INGREDIENTS

- ¼ cup red wine vinegar
- 1 teaspoon dried oregano (rub between hands to release oils)
- 2 cloves garlic, minced
- ½ teaspoon Dijon mustard
- 1 teaspoon salt
- ½ teaspoon pepper
- ½ cup extra-virgin olive oil

1. Measure the vinegar, oregano, garlic, mustard, salt, and pepper in a small bowl.

2. Whisk ingredients together and drizzle the olive oil into the bowl until emulsified.

Makes about 1 cup of dressing

Mustard Vinaigrette

INGREDIENTS

- 1 clove garlic, finely minced
- 1 tablespoon Dijon mustard
- 3 tablespoons balsamic vinegar
- 1 teaspoon soy or tamari sauce
- Salt and freshly ground black pepper to taste
- ½ cup extra-virgin olive oil

1. Combine all ingredients except the olive oil in a small mixing bowl.

2. Whisk ingredients together and drizzle the olive oil into the bowl until emulsified.

Makes about ½ cup of dressing

Creamy Soynnaise Dressing

INGREDIENTS

- ½ cup soynnaise
- 1 medium red bell pepper, minced
- ¼ cup raisins, chopped
- 1 tablespoon apple cider vinegar
- ¼ teaspoon curry powder

1. Combine all ingredients in a small bowl. Blend until well mixed.

2. Serve over cabbage slaw or torn lettuce.

Makes about ½ cup of dressing

Garlic Mustard Dressing

INGREDIENTS

- ½ head garlic
- ½ teaspoon Dijon mustard
- ¼ cup apple juice
- ¼ cup balsamic vinegar
- 2 tablespoons extra-light olive oil
- ½ teaspoon salt
- ⅛ teaspoon freshly ground black pepper

1. Preheat the oven to 400 degrees.

2. Slice 1 inch off the top of garlic so cloves are exposed; wrap the garlic in foil and roast until soft and fragrant, 40–45 minutes.

3. Allow the garlic to cool slightly and then squeeze the cloves into a mini-chopper or food processor.

4. Add the remaining ingredients; blend until smooth, adding more apple juice if necessary.

5. Store in the refrigerator for up to 7 days.

Makes about ½ cup of dressing

Classic Oil and Lemon Dressing

Consider this recipe to be like a blank canvas on which you will create your own work of art. Add the herbs and spices you enjoy to this base and then mix enough for several days. It keeps well when stored in an airtight container in the refrigerator.

INGREDIENTS

- 6 tablespoons extra-virgin olive oil
- 1½ tablespoons fresh lemon juice
- Herbs and spices of your choice (optional)
- Salt and freshly ground black pepper

1. Whisk together the oil and lemon juice until emulsified.

2. Add dried or fresh herbs and spices as you desire and whisk again. Season with salt and pepper to taste.

3. Pour over salad and toss.

Makes about 4 servings

Flatbread and Crackers

Leavening is not allowed on the Daniel Fast. However, unleavened bread such as matzo, chapatis, or tortillas can be enjoyed and offers a great complement to soups and salads.

You will also find recipes for corn chips and crackers in this section. Consider making these recipes in large batches and storing the foods in airtight containers for later use. Making crackers and flatbread can be a fun family project.

Chapatis or Indian Flatbread

Chapatis are similar to tortillas and are made with no baking powder. They are easy to make and keep well if stored in an airtight container. Chapatis are common in Southeast Asia and throughout Africa.

INGREDIENTS

- 2½ cups fine whole wheat flour (you can usually find this in the natural foods section of the supermarket or with the bulk foods)
- 1 pinch salt
- 2 cups water (or enough to make a soft dough)

1. Mix flour and salt in a large mixing bowl.

2. Make a hole in flour, add water, and use your hands to mix and make a soft dough.

3. Knead for 5 minutes, return to the bowl, cover with wet cloth, and refrigerate for 1 hour.

4. Heat a cast-iron skillet over medium-high heat until very hot.

5. Roll out half a handful of dough into a flat, round shape and place in pan, cooking for 1 minute on each side.

6. Once turned, press gently with a towel, until brown.

7. Repeat until all dough is used.

Makes 10 chapatis

Unleavened Bread

In my quest to find a recipe for bread that would be acceptable on the Daniel Fast, I found and tested this recipe for unleavened bread. This kind of bread has been around for thousands of years, and some scholars report that similar bread was baked on stones in the hot sun long before Christ's birth. The recipe takes a bit of extra time, but the bread is so healthy for you that you may use it all year long!

INGREDIENTS

- ½ cup olive oil
- ½ cup water
- Salt
- 2 cups whole wheat flour (regular or pastry grind)

1. Preheat the oven to 350 degrees.

2. In a large bowl, whisk together the olive oil, water, and salt until the mixture is frothy.

3. Stir in small portions of the flour, blending well and adding all the flour until the dough is the consistency of a cookie dough. Turn the dough onto a floured surface and knead with a quarter turn folding motion for about 5 minutes. Cover the dough with a kitchen towel and allow to rest for about 5 minutes.

4. Flour the surface again, and then roll the dough until it is the thickness of pie dough. Using a fork, make several pricks in the dough to allow air to release during baking. Cut the dough into squares in the size you desire (I like 2-inch squares, but larger pieces are fine).

5. Transfer the pieces to nonstick baking sheets or baking sheets lined with parchment paper.

6. Bake for about 8 to 10 minutes or until lightly browned. Adjust the baking time for crispier or softer bread.

Makes 6 servings

What Shape Do You Want?

This dough can be rolled flat and cut into squares, or you can also form a lump of dough into a flattened mound and then roll it into a round shape, similar to pie dough. Be sure to prick the dough with a fork so air can release during the baking.

Simple Matzo-Style Unleavened Bread

This recipe is similar to matzo bread, but kosher cooking engages many more elements than ingredients. However, this flour and water recipe is easy and makes a good addition to all your meals.

INGREDIENTS

- 2 cups whole wheat pastry flour
- Warm water

1. Preheat your oven to 450 degrees and line two large baking sheets with parchment paper.

2. Measure the flour into a large bowl; add water in small amounts and mix until you have a soft dough.

3. Turn the dough onto a floured surface and knead with a quarter turn folding motion for about 5 minutes. Cover the dough with a kitchen towel and allow to rest for about 5 minutes.

4. Break off egg-sized portions of the dough and stretch as thinly as you can before rolling into oval slabs that are as thin as possible. Prick each oval with a fork.

5. Transfer the pieces to a baking sheet and place it in the oven; bake until crisp and buckled, about 3 minutes.

6. Cool and eat.

Makes 6 servings

Homemade Corn Chips

Families from the Southwest especially miss corn chips during the Daniel Fast. That's because most chips found in the grocery stores are deep fried, making them off-limits during the Daniel Fast. But here's a recipe for homemade corn chips that you can whip up in no time. They are easy to make . . . but be warned—you might have to fend off family members who will want to snack on them as soon as the chips come out of the oven.

INGREDIENTS

- 1 cup cornmeal
- 1 tablespoon oil
- ½ teaspoon salt
- ¾ cup boiling water (plus enough to make dough the proper consistency)

1. Preheat the oven to 400 degrees.

2. Mix the cornmeal, oil, salt, and water in a large mixing bowl.

3. Scoop 1 heaping measuring teaspoonful of the mixture and place it on a well-greased baking sheet. (Use plenty of oil, or they will stick.)

4. Moisten fingers and pat out very thin, or use the bottom of a glass (flour or moisten to keep from sticking).

5. Bake for about 10 minutes, and then sprinkle with salt.

Makes about 1 pound of chips

Homemade Crackers

Making crackers is quick, easy, and fun. They can be made with various seasonings and many different kinds of grain. Try cornmeal with chili powder, rye with caraway or dill seeds, or whole wheat with garlic powder. Experiment! If made from cornmeal, buckwheat, or other nongluten grains, they can safely be eaten by gluten-intolerant individuals. This recipe makes a semicrisp, dense cracker.

INGREDIENTS

- 1¼ cups whole wheat flour, divided (rye, buckwheat, or cornmeal can be substituted)
- ½ teaspoon salt
- 2 tablespoons canola oil or olive oil; more as needed
- 4 tablespoons water; add more as needed
- 1 teaspoon seasoning such as dried herbs, chili powder, garlic powder, onion powder, etc. (optional)

1. Preheat oven to 400 degrees.

2. Using a food processor, mix 1 cup of the flour, salt, optional seasonings or herbs, and oil.

3. Add 3 tablespoons water and mix well. Gradually add more water, blending after each addition, until the mixture forms a compact ball. If it seems too sticky to handle, add a little more flour.

4. Sprinkle your work surface (or a baking sheet–sized piece of parchment paper) with some of the remaining flour; then press and roll the dough to about ⅛-inch thickness, trying to get it fairly uniform. If the dough is too dry to roll out, return it to the food processor and add a little more water. If necessary to prevent sticking, dust your hands and the rolling pin with a little more flour.

5. Place the rolled-out dough on a baking sheet dusted with a little flour or cornmeal. (If you've used parchment paper, transfer dough and paper to baking sheet.)

6. Bake for 10 to 15 minutes, until light brown.

7. Cool and break into pieces. If making several batches, mix another while the first one bakes. You can reuse the parchment paper several times.

Makes about 1 pound of crackers

Dips and Salsas

Appetizers and snacks are a good way to fight off cravings and to nourish your body with wholesome foods. Serve spreads and dips on homemade crackers or chips or with cut-up fresh vegetables.

I make a lot of hummus and enjoy it with celery, red pepper strips, or sliced carrots. I also like making flavorful salsas and serving them with homemade corn chips or as a condiment with bean burgers.

Basic Hummus

Hummus is a Middle Eastern bean dip that is a standard in my house during the Daniel Fast. I serve it with sliced vegetables, chapatis, or homemade crackers. There are many varieties to create interesting flavors! This is the basic recipe.

INGREDIENTS

- 1 can (15 ounces) chickpeas, drained, but reserve the liquid
- 3–5 tablespoons lemon juice (depending on taste)
- 1½ tablespoons tahini (sesame seed paste)
- 2 cloves garlic, minced
- ½ teaspoon salt
- 2 tablespoons olive oil

1. Place the chickpeas, lemon juice, tahini, garlic, and salt in a blender or food processor. Add ¼ cup of reserved liquid from canned chickpeas. Blend 3–5 minutes on low until thoroughly mixed and smooth.

2. Transfer the mixture to a serving bowl and create a shallow well in the center of the hummus. Add 1–2 tablespoons of olive oil in the well and gently blend.

3. Garnish with parsley (optional). Serve immediately with raw vegetables, homemade crackers, or flatbread.

Makes about 4 servings

Restaurant Style Hummus

This tasty recipe has some slight variations and calls for canned chickpeas, which makes it possible to whip this dip up in a few minutes. But you can use dried chickpeas if you prefer, following the directions on the package for cooking. The cayenne pepper adds some heat to the otherwise moderate flavor.

INGREDIENTS

- 3 tablespoons fresh lemon juice
- ¼ cup water
- 6 tablespoons tahini, stirred well
- 2 tablespoons extra-virgin olive oil, plus extra for drizzling
- 1 can (15 ounces) chickpeas, drained and rinsed
- 1 clove garlic, minced
- ½ teaspoon salt
- ¼ teaspoon ground cumin
- Pinch cayenne pepper
- 1 tablespoon minced fresh cilantro

1. Using a small bowl, combine the lemon juice and water.

2. In a separate small bowl, whisk together the tahini and 2 tablespoons oil.

3. Set aside 2 tablespoons chickpeas for garnish and process the remaining chickpeas, garlic, salt, cumin, and cayenne pepper in food processor until almost fully ground, about 15 seconds.

4. Scrape down bowl with rubber spatula. With the food processor still running, add lemon juice–water mixture in steady stream through feed tube. Scrape down bowl and continue to process for 1 minute.

5. Again, with the food processor still running, add oil-tahini mixture in a steady stream through feed tube; continue to process until hummus is smooth and creamy, about 15 seconds, scraping down bowl as needed.

6. Transfer hummus to serving bowl, sprinkle reserved chickpeas and cilantro over surface, cover with plastic wrap, and let stand until flavors meld, at least 30 minutes.

7. Drizzle with olive oil and serve.

Makes about 2 cups

Time-Saving Tip

You can also make this recipe up to five days ahead. Refrigerate the hummus and the garnishes separately; then, just before serving, stir in about 1 tablespoon of warm water if the texture is too thick. Add your garnishes, and serve.

White Bean Dip

This dip works well with sliced vegetables, crackers, or chips. It's easy to make and lasts several days if refrigerated.

INGREDIENTS

- 2 cans (15 ounces each) white beans, rinsed and drained
- 2 tablespoons roasted garlic
- 3 tablespoons extra-virgin olive oil
- 3 tablespoons freshly squeezed lemon juice
- Salt and pepper
- ¼ cup parsley leaves, to garnish

1. In a food processor, combine the beans, roasted garlic, olive oil, and lemon juice and process until smooth.

2. Season to taste with salt and pepper.

3. Garnish with fresh parsley leaves and serve with your favorite vegetables.

Makes 6–8 servings

Black Bean Dip

Similar to the white bean dip, this black bean dip is also wonderful served as an appetizer with sliced vegetables or homemade crackers or chips.

INGREDIENTS

- 1 plum tomato, diced
- 2 tablespoons diced red onion
- 1 tablespoon cilantro, chopped, plus sprigs for garnish
- 2 cans (15 ounces each) black beans, drained
- 1 tablespoon ground cumin
- 2 teaspoons hot sauce
- Salt

1. Place the tomato, onion, and cilantro into the bowl of a food processor and pulse until well chopped.

2. Add the black beans, cumin, hot sauce, and salt, to taste, and pulse until the mixture is mostly smooth.

3. Scrape into a bowl and garnish with cilantro sprigs. Serve with vegetables or chips.

Makes about 2 cups of dip

Black Bean and Mango Salsa

This is a Caribbean-inspired salsa and is great served with chapatis or corn chips as a snack or appetizer, or to go along with your dinner menu. You can also serve the salsa as a salad on lettuce leaves fashioned into edible bowls.

INGREDIENTS

- 1 cup black beans, home-cooked or canned
- 2 mangos, peeled, seeded, and finely diced
- ½ medium red bell pepper, cored, seeded, and finely diced
- ½ medium green bell pepper, cored, seeded, and finely diced
- ½ medium red onion, finely diced
- ¾ cup pineapple juice
- ½ cup fresh lime juice
- ½ cup chopped fresh cilantro leaves
- 2 tablespoons ground cumin
- 1 small jalapeño pepper, seeded and minced (use precaution when handling)
- Salt and freshly ground black pepper

1. As you prepare the ingredients, just place them in the same medium mixing bowl; gently blend and then adjust seasoning with salt and pepper to taste.

2. Cover with plastic wrap and refrigerate to blend the flavors, at least 1 hour or up to 4 days.

Makes about 5 cups

Homemade Guacamole

One of my personal favorites in the dip department is guacamole. The mild sweetness of the avocados combines well with other flavor-packed ingredients.

INGREDIENTS

- 3 avocados, ripe (I prefer Hass avocados because they seem to have more flavor.)
- 2 tablespoons minced onion
- 1 clove garlic, minced
- 1 small jalapeño pepper, minced (use precaution when handling)
- ¼ cup minced fresh cilantro leaves
- ¼ teaspoon table salt
- ½ teaspoon ground cumin (optional)
- 2 tablespoons lime juice
- Salt to taste

1. Prepare the minced ingredients first so they are ready to mix with the avocados as soon as they are cut.

2. Halve one avocado, remove pit, and scoop flesh into medium bowl. Mash flesh lightly with onion, garlic, jalapeño, cilantro, salt, and cumin (if using) with tines of a fork until just combined.

3. Halve and pit remaining two avocados, dicing them with skins on. Sprinkle lime juice over the diced avocado pieces before adding them to the mashed avocado mixture.

4. Mix entire contents of bowl lightly with fork until combined but still chunky. Adjust seasoning with salt, if necessary, and serve. (Guacamole can be covered with plastic wrap, pressed directly onto surface of mixture, and refrigerated up to one day. Return guacamole to room temperature, removing plastic wrap at the last moment before serving.)

Makes about 3 cups

Spicy Tomato Salsa

You can make this recipe ahead and then serve it a few times over the next several days. I like to serve this salsa with raw vegetables, including slices of carrot, cucumber, or jicama. I also like to fill celery stalks with the salsa for a crunchy treat.

INGREDIENTS

- 3 large tomatoes, diced small
- ½ cup tomato juice
- 1 chipotle chile, minced
- 1 red onion, diced small
- 1 clove garlic, minced
- ½ cup loosely packed, chopped fresh cilantro leaves
- ½ cup fresh lime juice
- Salt and pepper

1. Combine the tomatoes, tomato juice, chile, red onion, and garlic in a medium bowl.
2. Add the cilantro, lime juice, salt, and pepper in small amounts until you reach your desired taste.
3. Cover and refrigerate to fuse flavors, at least 1 hour or up to 5 days.

Makes about 5 cups

Chipotle What?

If you're not accustomed to cooking Mexican food, you may not be familiar with chipotle chiles. These delightful "heaters" are smoked jalapeño peppers and add a nice smoky flavor to this recipe. You can substitute other peppers if you prefer.

Black Bean and Corn Salsa

I love this recipe, not only because of the great flavors, but also because the colors are so bright and appetizing. Use this as a salsa with chips or vegetables. I like it best as a surprising punch in tofu scrambles.

INGREDIENTS

- 1 can (15 ounces) black beans, rinsed and drained
- 1 can (15 ounces) whole kernel corn, drained

- 1 teaspoon minced fresh jalapeño pepper (use precaution when handling)
- 2 Roma tomatoes, seeded and chopped
- 1 red bell pepper, seeded and cut in small dices
- ⅓ cup chopped fresh cilantro
- ¼ cup diced red onion
- ¼ cup fresh lime juice
- 1 teaspoon salt
- 1 avocado, diced
- Homemade corn chips (see recipe on page 200)

1. Combine all ingredients in a large bowl except for the avocado and chips; toss lightly until well blended.

2. Cover and chill for at least two hours, then add avocado just before serving.

3. Serve with homemade corn chips or with sliced vegetables.

Makes 4–6 servings

Black Olive Tapenade

Tapenade is simple to make and a flavorful relish or spread for an appetizer. You can serve it with crackers or chips, but using jicama slices (jicama is a root vegetable that has a consistency of a raw potato or pear) is a good way to increase your vegetable servings and save on calories.

INGREDIENTS

- 20 pitted kalamata olives, coarsely chopped
- 1 tablespoon capers, rinsed, drained, and chopped
- 1 teaspoon fresh lemon juice
- 2 teaspoons extra-virgin olive oil
- Freshly ground black pepper to taste

1. Combine olives, capers, lemon juice, and olive oil in a bowl.

2. Season to taste with freshly ground black pepper.

3. Serve with sliced jicama, chips, or crackers; store in airtight container in refrigerator for up to 30 days.

Makes 4 servings

Snacks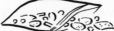

Eating two small snacks during the day not only helps fend off cravings, but research shows it helps with weight loss and digestion. The trick is to keep snacks in proportionate amounts rather than meal-size servings. For example, a snack-size portion of raw almonds is ¼ cup or about ten almonds.

I measure snack-size servings of nuts into small ziplock bags. I keep a few bags in my car for those times when hunger calls and I'm away from home.

Roasted Chickpeas

This is a crunchy, nutlike snack and a great alternative to oily and fattening chips.

INGREDIENTS

- 4 cups cooked or canned chickpeas
- ½ teaspoon salt
- 4 tablespoons olive oil

1. Preheat the oven to 375 degrees.
2. Drain and pat the chickpeas dry with paper towels. Mix the salt and oil together in a large bowl; add the chickpeas, and toss until well coated.
3. Spread the chickpeas on heavy-weight baking sheets in a single layer.
4. Roast for 45 minutes, stirring every 15 minutes, being careful not to burn the chickpeas.
5. The chickpeas are done when they are golden brown and completely dried with no chewy centers. If they are underdone, roast longer, checking every 5 minutes and stirring.
6. Allow to cool and then store in an airtight container.

Makes 4–6 servings

Roasted Kidney Beans

Most people don't even think of using beans as a snack. But here is another great recipe that serves as an excellent alternative to fattening nuts and chips.

INGREDIENTS

- 6 cups dried, whole kidney beans, soaked for at least 8 hours
- 1 large onion, quartered
- 2 stalks celery, cut into large chunks

- 3 tablespoons olive oil
- Salt and spices

1. After soaking the kidney beans, place them in a large pot and cook them in fresh water with the onion and celery. Drain and discard the onion and celery.
2. Coat a cookie sheet with the olive oil and then toss the beans in the olive oil until well coated.
3. Slow roast the beans in the oven at 200 degrees for 4 to 8 hours. Remove from the oven when crunchy and toss in salt and spices.

Makes 6 cups

How the Bean Growers Cook Beans
Place washed beans into a large pot or Dutch oven and cover with 6 cups fresh water for each pound (2 cups) of beans, or to about 1 inch above the beans. Add 1 to 2 tablespoons oil (to prevent boiling over) and seasonings as desired. Boil gently with lid tilted until tender when tasted, 1½ to 2 hours. Add hot water as needed to keep beans just covered with liquid. The best rule is to test frequently during cooking and then come to your own decision when beans are tender and taste "done."

—Central Bean Company[12]

Crunchy Kale Chips

I found this recipe and was amazed at the guiltless delight these chips embody. Light, crunchy, and salty, these chips are a wonderful alternative to the deep-fried chips that pack the pounds on our hips and cholesterol in our bloodstreams!

INGREDIENTS
- 6 cups kale, about 2 bunches, rinsed, with stems removed
- 1 tablespoon apple cider vinegar
- 2 tablespoons olive oil
- 2 teaspoons salt (This makes them pretty salty. You may want to reduce the amount and then sprinkle the chips with salt.)

1. Preheat the oven to 350 degrees.
2. Cut the kale leaves into 2- to 3-inch pieces.
3. Combine the vinegar, oil, and salt in a large bowl; add the kale and toss them by hand to make sure all the leaves are coated.

4. Place the leaves in a single layer on baking sheets (I like to use parchment paper for easy cleanup) and bake until they are crispy, about 20 minutes. If the kale leaves are not sizzling a bit or getting a little crispy, turn up the heat to 400 degrees.

5. Time for baking varies depending on the size of your chips and desired crispness. The outer edges cook quicker than the pieces from near the stem.

Makes 8 servings

Cutting the Kale

I find it easiest to use kitchen shears to cut the stems from the kale. I make a V-cut into the kale leaf and remove the tougher stems. It's an easy and fast method!

New Popcorn Snacks

Pull out the popcorn popper and make a tasty snack for you and your family. The recipes here call for unpopped popcorn. Most microwave varieties include ingredients that are not allowed on the Daniel Fast. However, more and more food manufacturers are catching on that people don't want chemicals added to their food. So check out the ingredients on the label if you are considering using microwave popcorn for these recipes.

New Spicy Popcorn Snack

INGREDIENTS

- 1 cup popcorn kernels
- 2 tablespoons vegetable oil
- ½ teaspoon sweet paprika
- 1 teaspoon salt
- ½ teaspoon garlic powder
- 1 teaspoon cumin
- ¼ teaspoon cayenne pepper
- Olive oil cooking spray

1. Pop the corn using an air popper; or heat the vegetable oil in a pan over medium-high heat; add corn and cover, shaking pan often.

2. Meanwhile, blend the spices in a small bowl until well mixed.

3. When the corn is popped, transfer to a large bowl and spray with olive oil; sprinkle with spice mix and toss to distribute among the popped kernels.

Makes about 8 servings

New Spicy Curry Peanut Popcorn

I'll warn you that this snack is messy to make, but fun for kids and steeped in spicy flavors.

INGREDIENTS

- ½ cup popcorn kernels
- 2 tablespoons vegetable oil (eliminate if you use an air popper)
- 2 tablespoons creamy peanut butter (made only with 100% peanuts and with or without salt)
- 1 teaspoon curry powder
- 1 teaspoon chili paste

1. Pop the corn using an air popper; or heat the oil in a pan over medium-high heat; add popcorn and cover, shaking pan often.

2. Transfer popcorn to a large bowl.

3. Place the peanut butter, curry powder, and chili paste in a small bowl; heat in microwave for 30 seconds; stir to blend well. If the sauce is too stiff, add a little hot water to make it thick and creamy.

4. Carefully drizzle the hot peanut butter sauce over the popcorn; using two wooden spoons or your hands with food-grade gloves, gently mix the popcorn with the sauce and form into small clusters.

Makes 8 servings

New Rice Cake Snacks

You may need to look in the natural foods section of your supermarket to find rice cakes that don't include chemicals or sweeteners. My favorites are those made with brown rice and just a little salt. I stock up when they're on sale and enjoy them with a variety of toppings.

INGREDIENTS

- 2 rice cakes (made from brown rice)
- 2 tablespoons peanut butter
- ¼ cup raisins

1. Spread each of the rice cakes with peanut butter.

2. Top with raisins and serve.

Makes 1 or 2 servings

Variations:

- Add sliced bananas, chopped nuts, and/or shaved fresh ginger.
- Spread the rice cake with hummus, and top with a fresh salsa.
- Spread the rice cake with mashed avocado and top with a slice of tomato and lettuce.
- Use your imagination: let the rice cake be your canvas and Daniel Fast–friendly ingredients your "paint."

New Snack Packs

Okay, I'm guilty as charged! There are times when I'm in my car or out running errands and I start craving certain foods. So I started creating my own little snack packs, which come to my rescue when hunger pangs start. I keep a supply in my car and in my cupboard. Making my own snack packs saves money and helps with portion control.

INGREDIENTS

- 1 pack of snack-sized ziplock plastic bags

A variety of snacks of your choice that comply with the Daniel Fast food lists, measured in single portions. Ideas for snack-pack ingredients include:

- Almonds
- Daniel Fast Trail Mix (see recipe on next page)
- Dried fruit
- Peanuts
- Raisins
- Sunflower seeds
- Crackers (be sure to review the ingredients if you purchase crackers)
- Walnuts (my favorite)

1. Place a single-portion serving of a snack item in each bag and seal.
2. Place all the bags in an airtight container or into a larger ziplock bag to ensure freshness.
3. Stash the snacks in your cupboard, car, lunch sack, desk drawer, or wherever you might need them.

New Daniel Fast Trail Mix

Keep a supply of this healthy snack around the house for you and your family during the Daniel Fast and even when you're not fasting. Use the ingredients below to make a batch or as a guideline to customize the recipe to your liking. There are lots of possibilities—just make sure all items are consistent with the Daniel Fast food lists.

INGREDIENTS

- ½ cup chopped dried apricots and/or dried pears
- ½ cup chopped dried apples and/or prunes
- ½ cup raisins or chopped dates
- 1½ cups raw sunflower seeds and/or raw pumpkin seeds
- 1 cup unsalted nuts (peanuts, walnuts, and/or almonds)

1. Mix all the ingredients in a large bowl.

2. Store in an airtight container.

Makes 4 cups of trail mix

New Veggie and Fruit Snacks

Another way to set yourself and your family members up for success during your Daniel Fast is to keep appetizing fruits and vegetables available and prepared. I do best when I wash, peel, and pare all my produce as soon as I return from the grocery store. Consider making little snack packs with fruits and veggies for school and work lunches, after-school snacks, and other times during the day. This may be a new practice that can develop into a healthy discipline that you continue long after the fast.

INGREDIENTS

- Apples	- Mango	- Strawberries
- Bananas	- Papaya	- Melon
- Carrots	- Pea pods	- Oranges
- Celery	- Pears	- Tomatoes
- Cherries	- Radishes	- Green beans
- Cucumber	- Sweet peppers	- Broccoli
- Grapes	- Blueberries	- Cauliflower

- The ideas for how to serve these natural treats are endless. You can create platters with mixed veggies and homemade hummus for dipping.

- Have fun with your children! Lay out an array of fresh fruits and vegetables; give each child a large paper plate and let them create a face using the vegetables. (Of course, the plan is that they eat the items after they've shared their artwork with the others!)
- Serve fruits and vegetables along with your main dish instead of a salad.
- Serve fresh fruit as dessert.

Condiments and Extras

Another challenge you might face during the Daniel Fast is finding condiments that meet the permissible ingredients criteria. Again, making your own is often the best and least expensive solution.

You will find recipes for soynnaise (mayonnaise made from soy products) and sweetener-free ketchup in this section. I find them very satisfying, and I love that they only have a few calories in each serving.

Soy Milk Soynnaise ("Mayonnaise")

It is so easy to make mayonnaise from soy milk that I never buy it anymore. Use this homemade soynnaise just as you would use traditional mayonnaise.

INGREDIENTS

- ½ cup soy milk
- 2 tablespoons fresh lemon juice
- Sea salt to taste (start with a pinch and add more as needed)
- 1 tablespoon cider vinegar
- ½ cup canola or olive oil

1. Put the soy milk, lemon juice, vinegar, and salt into a blender and blend well.

2. While still blending, add the oil in a slow, steady stream.

3. Continue to blend until the soynnaise becomes creamy, about 5 minutes.

4. Adjust seasoning and be creative by adding herbs and spices at this stage. Blend only until well mixed.

5. Store in airtight container in the refrigerator.

Makes about 1 cup

More or Less . . .

You can increase or decrease this recipe but keep the amount of soy milk and oil the same: 1 cup soy milk, then 1 cup oil. The other ingredients can be altered to your liking.

Tofu Soynnaise ("Mayonnaise")

As you know, regular mayonnaise is made with eggs, which are not allowed on the Daniel Fast. This mayo is okay for fasting and all year long.

INGREDIENTS

- 1 cup cubed soft tofu
- 4 tablespoons olive oil
- 3 teaspoons fresh lemon juice
- 1 teaspoon apple juice concentrate
- ¼ teaspoon sea salt

1. Place the tofu, olive oil, lemon juice, apple juice, and salt in a blender. Cover and blend until smooth.

2. Store in an airtight container in the refrigerator.

Makes 1 cup

Strawberry Soynnaise Dip or Salad Dressing

Serve this strawberry soynnaise as a dip with vegetables or fruit. Try it with carrot sticks, blanched broccoli spears, lightly cooked asparagus, whole strawberries, banana slices, and pineapple chunks. For a bolder taste, add a little minced garlic.

INGREDIENTS

- ½ cup soynnaise
- ¼ cup crushed strawberries

1. Mix the soynnaise with the crushed strawberries and serve as a dip or a dressing.

Makes ¾ cup serving

Daniel Fast Ketchup

Here is a quick recipe for homemade ketchup with no sugar.

INGREDIENTS

- 1 cup tomato paste
- 2 cups tomato sauce
- 2 tablespoons apple juice
- 1 teaspoon kosher salt
- ¼ teaspoon ground cloves
- ⅛ teaspoon ground allspice

1. Place the tomato paste, tomato sauce, apple juice, salt, cloves, and allspice in a large saucepan and blend. Bring to a boil over medium heat; then reduce the heat to low and simmer, uncovered, until thickened, about 20 minutes.

2. Spoon into airtight container and store in refrigerator.

Makes about 3 cups

Daniel Fast Ketchup from Fresh Tomatoes

INGREDIENTS

- 4½ pounds ripe tomatoes, seeded and roughly chopped
- 2 tablespoons apple juice (or more to achieve desired flavor)
- 2 yellow onions, roughly chopped
- ½ cup lightly packed celery leaves
- ½ cup distilled white vinegar
- 1 teaspoon kosher salt
- 1 bay leaf
- ¼ teaspoon ground cloves
- ⅛ teaspoon ground allspice

1. Place the tomatoes, apple juice, onions, celery leaves, vinegar, salt, bay leaf, cloves, and allspice in a large saucepan and blend. Bring to a boil over medium heat; then reduce heat to low and simmer, uncovered, until thickened, about 3 hours.

2. Adjust the seasoning and sweetness. Discard the bay leaf and place ¼ of the ketchup in a blender or food processor; cover and process until smooth. Pour through strainer and repeat until all the ketchup is strained.

3. Spoon into airtight containers and store in the refrigerator.

Makes about 4 cups

New Garam Masala

This spice blend is particularly popular in northern India and other south Asian countries. *Garam* is translated as "hot," but that refers to the pungency of the spices rather than its kick. *Masala* means "mixture" or "blend." So this is a blend of spices that produce a very flavorful result. It's likely that you have all the ingredients to make garam masala in your own collection of spices. Blending it yourself allows you to adjust the flavors or even add other spices if you desire.

INGREDIENTS

- 1 tablespoon ground cumin
- 1½ teaspoons ground coriander
- 1½ teaspoons ground cardamom
- 1½ teaspoons ground pepper
- 1 teaspoon ground cinnamon
- ½ teaspoon ground ginger
- ½ teaspoon ground cloves
- ½ teaspoon ground nutmeg

1. Place all the ingredients in a bowl. Mix until well blended.

2. Store in an airtight container and use in soups, stews, casseroles, etc.

New Cashew Butter

This great alternative to peanut butter can also be used in recipes to make dressings and sauces creamy. Be sure to use whole cashews that have been kept in sealed containers since the nut can quickly turn rancid, due to its high oil content.

INGREDIENTS

- 2 cups unsalted, whole cashews (preferably raw)
- 2 or more tablespoons vegetable oil
- ¼ teaspoon salt

1. Combine the nuts, 2 tablespoons of the oil, and salt in a food processor or blender; blend on high speed for about 30 seconds.

2. Use a spatula to scrape down the sides of the container; process again until the cashew butter is smooth.

3. Add additional oil in small amounts to reach the desired consistency.

4. Store the cashew butter in an airtight container in the refrigerator until you are ready to add it to your recipes, or use it as an alternative to peanut butter.

Makes about 2 cups

Note: This same process can be used to make homemade peanut butter.

New Cashew Cream

More and more people are using cashew cream as an alternative to dairy cream. It's a particularly good option when you're on the Daniel Fast and have a recipe that calls for cream. Be sure to use fresh, whole, raw cashews for best results. You can keep the cashew cream in the refrigerator and use as needed. You can also freeze cashew cream, which is best used within six months.

INGREDIENTS

- 2 cups whole raw cashews (not pieces, which are often dry), rinsed very well under cold water
- Water as directed

1. Put cashews in a bowl with enough cold water to cover them. Cover bowl and refrigerate overnight.

2. Drain the cashews and rinse with fresh cool water.

3. Place the cashews in a food processor or blender; add enough fresh cold water just to cover the nuts; blend on high for several minutes until very smooth.

4. This will create a thick cream that can be used in recipes for soups, stews, dressings, and more. If you need a lighter cream, add more water and process the mixture

5. Cream will keep in refrigerator for several days.

Makes about 1¼ cups

New Faux Feta Cheese

Use this substitute for feta cheese in salads or with pasta. It's best to make it the day before, though that's not necessary if you don't have the time. It's great to keep on hand to sprinkle over salad recipes included in this book.

INGREDIENTS

- ¼ cup olive oil
- ¼ cup water
- ½ cup apple cider vinegar
- 2 teaspoons salt
- 1 tablespoon dried basil
- 1 teaspoon dried oregano
- ½ teaspoon dried onion
- ½ teaspoon pepper
- Pinch of dried hot pepper flakes
- 1 pound firm tofu, herb flavored; cubed or crumbled

1. Whisk together all ingredients but tofu in a bowl.

2. Add tofu and stir. Let sit for at least an hour.

Makes about a pound of faux feta cheese

Daniel Fast Menus

SAMPLE MENUS

Day	Breakfast	Lunch	Dinner	Snack
1	Muesli with soy milk Sliced fruit	Steamed vegetables with brown rice Apple	Susan's Vegetarian Chili Green salad Orange slices	Hummus with vegetable plate
2	Drew's Breakfast Burritos	Susan's Vegetarian Chili Carrot and celery sticks	Bean Burgers with Black Bean and Mango Salsa Green salad Apple slices	Fruit plate Almonds
3	Apple Pie Oatmeal with soy milk Apple slices	Plentiful Vegetable Soup Salad greens with vinaigrette	Tex-Mex Chili Pot Red, Black, and Yellow Delight Salad Fruit plate	White Bean Dip with carrots and celery

Day	Breakfast	Lunch	Dinner	Snack
4	Berry Banana Smoothie Raw almonds	Moroccan Vegetarian Stew Green salad Sliced apple	Tangy Bean and Spinach Salad Kirsten's Favorite Yellow Rice Apple slices	Fruit kabobs
5	Dried Fruit and Almond Granola with soy milk Sliced banana	Lentil Soup Celery with peanut butter	Daniel Fast Cabbage Rolls Fruit kabobs	Black Bean Dip with carrot slices
6	Tofu-Veggie Breakfast Scramble Orange slices	Classic Navy Bean Soup Green salad Fresh orange	Turkish Salad Plentiful Vegetable Soup	Herb-Roasted Sweet Potato Fries
7	Oatmeal with soy milk Sliced banana	Tex-Mex Chili Pot Green salad Fresh apple	Curried Vegetables with Tofu Green salad Fruit platter	Hummus with vegetable plate
8	Yummy Brown Rice with Apple Sliced citrus fruit	Black Bean, Corn, and Brown Rice Stuffed Peppers Celery and carrot sticks	Quick Slow Cooker Veggie Soup Green salad Sliced orange	Vegetable plate with Tofu Soynnaise
9	Potato and Scallion Breakfast Frittata Fresh ruby grapefruit sections	Golden Carrot Soup Sweet Brown Rice with Spicy Sauce	Fast Food Stir-Fry Brown Rice with Vegetables Fruit plate	Fruit plate

Day	Breakfast	Lunch	Dinner	Snack
10	Four Grain Muesli with soy milk Sliced apples	Steamed vegetables with brown rice Apple	Bean Burgers with Salsa Curried Bean and Rice Salad Orange slices	White Bean Dip with carrots and celery
11	Berry Banana Smoothie Almonds or walnuts	Susan's Vegetarian Chili Carrot and celery sticks	Tuscan Villa Bean Soup Mixed green salad with garnishes	Fruit kabobs
12	Banana Wheat Bran Cereal with soy milk Sliced apple	Moo Shu Vegetables Indian Flatbread Apple	Susan's Vegetarian Chili Fresh Corn Salad	Vegetable plate Almonds or walnuts
13	Curried Tofu Scramble Orange slices	Daniel Fast Cabbage Soup Sliced fruit	Curried Vegetables with Tofu Fruit plate	Herb-Roasted Sweet Potato Fries
14	Tomato and Green Pepper Tofu Scramble Sliced fruit	Plentiful Vegetable Soup Salad greens with vinaigrette	Fast Food Stir-Fry Brown Rice with Vegetables Green salad Orange slices	Fruit plate
15	Strawberry Oatmeal Smoothie Sliced banana	Moroccan Vegetarian Stew Green salad	Susan's Vegetarian Chili Green salad Orange slices	White Bean Dip with carrots and celery

Day	Breakfast	Lunch	Dinner	Snack
16	Four Grain Muesli with soy milk Sliced apple	Lentil Soup Celery with peanut butter	Bean Burgers with Black Bean and Mango Salsa Green salad Apple slices	Fruit kabobs
17	East Indian Mango Lassi Smoothie Almonds or walnuts	Classic Navy Bean Soup Green salad Fresh orange	Tex-Mex Chili Pot Red, Black, and Yellow Delight Salad Fruit plate	Roasted Kidney Beans Sliced fruit
18	Curried Tofu Scramble Orange slices	Tex-Mex Chili Pot Green salad Fresh grapes	Tangy Bean and Spinach Salad Kirsten's Favorite Yellow Rice Sliced apple	Hummus with vegetable plate
19	Drew's Breakfast Burritos Orange slices	Black Bean, Corn, and Brown Rice Stuffed Peppers Celery and carrot sticks	Daniel Fast Cabbage Rolls Fruit kabobs	Vegetable Plate with Tofu Soynnaise
20	Banana Wheat Bran Cereal with soy milk Sliced apple	Basic Black Bean Soup Tomato Salad with Walnuts	Turkish Salad Plentiful Vegetable Soup	Fruit plate
21	Potato and Scallion Breakfast Frittata Fresh ruby grapefruit sections	Sweet Potato Salad Sliced apple	Popeye Burgers Green salad Fruit platter	Herb-Roasted Sweet Potato Fries with Tofu Soynnaise

MEAL PLANNING WORKSHEET

Here is a meal planning worksheet template. Remember that this is a spiritual fast. Simplicity and moderation are in order. Go to http://www.Daniel-Fast.com to print additional worksheets.

Day	Breakfast	Lunch	Dinner	Snacks

Twenty-One-Day
Daniel Fast Devotional

STUDIES INDICATE that there are 2.1 billion Christians on the earth today. That's a lot of people! Christianity is the largest of all the religions in the world and includes more than 20,800 denominations. That's a lot of churches! But I wonder how many of the individuals who call themselves Christians would also consider themselves to be *disciples* of Jesus Christ.

Why the distinction? Many people attend church; let's call them "church attendees." But a disciple is something different. A disciple of Christ is a student who learns and follows the Master's teachings and lives according to His way. When you follow Christ, it doesn't mean that you will consider or obey selected parts of His teaching and ignore others. No, a disciple takes His teaching as truth in its entirety and then shapes his or her life according to those truths.

I can say without wavering or qualification that I am a Christian; it's my label. But the mantle that covers me is that I am a disciple of Jesus Christ. It is Jesus and His teachings that shape my life, determine my future, and serve as the foundation on which I stand in all things.

As a disciple, I learn and study God's Word so I can discover more about how I am to live, serve, and behave. It's a lifelong process with immeasurable treasures of joy, knowledge, peace, and supernatural power.

My hope is that you, too, can call yourself a disciple of Jesus Christ. My prayer is that the following devotions stir up your faith and strengthen your walk with your Father as you experience the Daniel Fast. And for this reason I do not cease to pray for you . . .

And to ask that you may be filled with the knowledge of His will in all wisdom and spiritual understanding; that you may walk worthy of the Lord, fully pleasing Him, being fruitful in every good work and increasing in the knowledge of God; strengthened with all might, according to His glorious power, for all patience and longsuffering with joy; giving thanks to the Father who has qualified us to be partakers of the inheritance of the saints in the light. He has delivered us from the power of darkness and conveyed us into the kingdom of the Son of His love, in whom we have redemption through His blood, the forgiveness of sins.

He is the image of the invisible God, the firstborn over all creation. For by Him all things were created that are in heaven and that are on earth, visible and invisible, whether thrones or dominions or principalities or powers. All things were created through Him and for Him. And He is before all things, and in Him all things consist. And He is the head of the body, the church, who is the beginning, the firstborn from the dead, that in all things He may have the preeminence.

—COLOSSIANS 1:9-18

DAY 1

Firstfruits Offering

The best of all firstfruits of any kind, and every sacrifice of any kind from all your sacrifices, shall be the priest's; also you shall give to the priest the first of your ground meal, to cause a blessing to rest on your house. —Ezekiel 44:30

Today is the first day of your fast. You are stepping into a different experience of feeding your soul, strengthening your spirit, and renewing your body. By entering into this special period of time, you are consecrating yourself (setting yourself apart) to focus more intently on the Lord and His ways.

We don't hear much about firstfruit offerings anymore. But they were a customary part of life for Old Testament believers, and there are many ways to make firstfruit offerings today. In Ezekiel 44:30, we see that the firstfruit is for the priest. So on this first day of consecrated prayer and fasting, you can say to Jesus, your High Priest, "Lord, today I give You the first of me. I put You first in my life."

We are also asked to give a firstfruits offering of our resources, just as God instructed the Israelites to do with their produce. The promised reward was "a blessing to rest on your house." You will recall that both Cain and Abel gave offerings to the Lord. Abel gave the firstborn of his flock and it pleased the Lord. But Cain's heart was not right before the Lord. Scholars conclude that his offering was not the best he had to offer, but rather leftovers. God rejected this offering.

The Lord doesn't want our spare time or our leftover efforts. He wants to be first in our lives. He wants the best of us. Throughout Scripture we are commanded to put God first. Exodus 20:5 says, "You shall not bow down to them nor serve them. For I, the LORD your God, am a jealous God." And in Matthew 6:33, "But seek first the kingdom of God and His righteousness, and all these things shall be added to you."

When we put God first in our lives, when He is the first and last authority in all that we do, then we are pleasing to the Lord and we have access to all He has for us. Psalm 103:1-2 says it beautifully: "Bless the LORD, O my soul; and all that is within me, bless His holy name! Bless the LORD, O my soul, and forget not all His benefits."

Does God want this position of priority because He craves our attention or needs our admiration? Maybe in part. I believe the underlying reason that God wants us to put Him first in our lives is because of the amazing, powerful, and immeasurable love He has for each one of us. He wants to pour out His mercy, grace, goodness, wisdom, and blessing over us in abundance. He wants us to be all He created us to be so we can experience a marvelous life and accomplish the good works He has already assigned to us.

The greatness He has planned for each of us is so enormous that the only way it can be fully realized is for us to stay close to Him. Likewise, His love and care are so deep and so broad and He desires to have an intimate and loving relationship with each of us that we must be close to Him to share in that bond. Finally, we know that our adversary the devil walks about like a roaring lion, seeking whom he may devour. His goal is to steal, kill, and destroy us, and we need the protection and counsel of our Father and His forces, available to defend us and realize the victory.

Do you hear the Holy Spirit's still, small voice beckoning you to come closer? Is God calling you to make adjustments in your life so that He is first in every area? Your period of prayer and fasting is a perfect time to hear the Lord and discover how much He desires you and every aspect of your life. Open your heart to Him and seek His wisdom and counsel. He will instruct you and guide you as you draw closer to Him and His ways. His arms are open wide, so respond to His warm and gracious invitation and come.

DAY 2

Sanctified by Truth

They are not of the world, just as I am not of the world. Sanctify them by Your truth. Your word is truth. As You sent Me into the world, I also have sent them into the world. —JOHN 17:16-18

Not long before Jesus started the journey toward His crucifixion, He talked to the Father about us. As our Advocate, He prayed for us even before He was sitting at the right hand of God. He was pleading our case and asking our Creator to bless us and keep us. One of those prayers was, "Sanctify them by Your truth."

The Greek word for "sanctify" is *hagiazo*, and it means "to make holy, purify, or consecrate." *Consecrate* means "to make full, to fulfill a calling, and to set apart for a holy purpose."

So in John 17:16-18 Jesus is saying to our Father, "These people are different now, Father. They're more like Me and not like the rest of the world. So please make them holy, pure, and able to fulfill Your calling on their lives through Your truth. Because just as You sent Me into the world to do Your business, I have sent them into the world to do Your business."

You and I are people set apart with a commission from Christ to do the business of God, which is to reconcile the world to Him. He has equipped us with unseen powers and tools to accomplish this task. He's given us everything we need. We are His army, His chosen people.

One of the important elements of fasting is consecration. We are consecrating this time and our lives unto the Lord. It is different from our normal, everyday routine. We are setting ourselves apart. In the Roman Catholic Church, priests, nuns, and monks are consecrated for religious service. Church buildings are consecrated or dedicated for spiritual purposes, similar to the Tabernacle in Jewish life. Furnishings in the Tabernacle were consecrated, set apart for spiritual practices. Belshazzar, the king of Babylon when Daniel was still a captive, unwittingly put his life in jeopardy when he drank from something that God had intended for a holy purpose:

> *Then they brought the gold vessels that had been taken from the temple of the house of God which had been in Jerusalem; and the king and his lords, his wives, and his concubines drank from them. They drank wine, and praised the gods of gold and silver, bronze and iron, wood and stone. In the same hour the fingers of a man's hand appeared and wrote opposite the lampstand on the plaster of the wall of the king's palace; and the king saw the part of the hand that wrote.* —DANIEL 5:3-5

Because of the king's brazen action, Daniel was summoned to read the writing on the wall, which warned of the doom that was to come to the king and to his nation. The king was slain that night, and the kingdom of Babylon soon began to crumble.

Another word closely associated with consecration is *sanctification*, which means "to be set apart for spiritual or holy purposes." When God led the captive Israelites out of Egypt, He said to them, "I will take you as My people, and I will be your God" (Exodus 6:7). He called the Jews to separate themselves from others in the world and to focus their lives on Him. He gave them innumerable promises for a good life if they would put Him first and follow His ways.

In John 17:16-18, Jesus is praying to the Father asking that we be sanctified, set aside for a holy purpose. And how will we be sanctified? By the truth that is in the Word of God.

As you continue on your fast, think about ways the Lord is calling you to be separate from the world. Ask the Holy Spirit to show you areas in your life that you could realign in order to be consistent with God's Word. Remember that you are a chosen person with a purpose to fulfill the business of God. Then set your mind to follow that call, to submit yourself to the Lord, and to walk in His ways.

DAY 3

What Do You Want Jesus to Do for You?

Jesus answered and said to him, "What do you want Me to do for you?" —MARK 10:51

As I read the Scriptures I like to picture the scene in my imagination so I can glean more truth from the Word. That's what I did when I was reading Mark 10. The story about the blind man, Bartimaeus, is told in just seven verses (46-52), yet it's packed with powerful truths we can use today.

Now they came to Jericho. As [Jesus] went out of Jericho with His disciples and a great multitude, blind Bartimaeus, the son of Timaeus, sat by the road begging. And when he heard that it was Jesus of Nazareth, he began to cry out and say, "Jesus, Son of David, have mercy on me!"

Then many warned him to be quiet; but he cried out all the more, "Son of David, have mercy on me!" So Jesus stood still and commanded him to be called. Then they called the blind man, saying to him, "Be of good cheer. Rise, He is calling you." And throwing aside his garment, he rose and came to Jesus.

So Jesus answered and said to him, "What do you want Me to do for you?"

The blind man said to Him, "Rabboni, that I may receive my sight."

Then Jesus said to him, "Go your way; your faith has made you well." And immediately he received his sight and followed Jesus on the road. —MARK 10:46-52

Blind Bartimaeus had a critical need. It was the hardship in his life that gave him the most grief and kept him trapped as a beggar. Bartimaeus knew about Jesus' reputation so when he learned that He was about to pass him by, he called out to Him. Bartimaeus knew and trusted Jesus as the Healer, even though he had never seen or talked to Him before. He had faith in who Jesus was and what Jesus could accomplish.

Here we are today in a similar situation. We, too, have hardships in our lives. Perhaps it's an illness, financial pressures, or marital problems. We, too, can call out to Jesus for help . . . but we also need to *know* who He is, even though we have never seen Him with our own eyes.

As Bartimaeus cried out, those around him tried to get him to be quiet. This can happen in our circumstances as well. Family members, friends, and church traditions can try to keep us from relying on Jesus to meet our needs. Sometimes the things that try to quiet us are more subtle, like intellect, unbelief, or fear. But like Bartimaeus, we must ignore these "voices" and cry out all the more.

It's interesting that as soon as Jesus gave His attention to Bartimaeus, all those around Him changed their tune! They moved from being critics to observers and witnesses.

When Bartimaeus got the message that Jesus was calling for him, he threw off his garment and went to Jesus. The garment has significance. It was a beggar's cloak that the authorities provided to needy people. The cloak gave them the right to beg and showed others that their calamities made them worthy of the givers' donations. But Bartimaeus tossed his beggar's garment away even before he received his sight.

Then Jesus asked him, "What do you want Me to do for you?" I find that question very interesting. It was obvious that Bartimaeus was blind. So why did Jesus not just heal him? I think this question was to test Bartimaeus's faith. He could have asked Jesus for money or for food. That would be the typical request of a beggar. But instead, Bartimaeus demonstrated his faith in Christ's ability to heal him and asked for the impossible: "Rabboni, that I may receive my sight."

Jesus responded to the request by saying, "Go your way; your faith has made you well." This is so powerful. How many times do we beg Jesus to move and perform a miracle for us? Yet here, Jesus says that it was Bartimaeus's faith that gave him his sight. There is no indication that Jesus touched him or prayed to the Father for the miracle. Instead, Jesus said that it was Bartimaeus's faith that made him well.

Bartimaeus knew Jesus healed. He activated his faith by calling out to Jesus even when all the voices surrounding him told him to be quiet. He threw off the garment that marked him as a blind man, and he told Jesus exactly what he wanted and knew Jesus could give him. And then the impossible happened!

What are the problems in your life today? What do you want Jesus to do for you? And what do you need to do to *know* Jesus, to activate your faith, and to expect the impossible?

Jesus is calling to you, just like He called to Bartimaeus. Do you hear Him? What voices are drowning out His beckoning? Step out in faith—and receive what the Lord wants you to have today.

DAY 4

Five Smooth Stones

> *David fastened his sword to his armor and tried to walk, for he had not tested them. And David said to Saul, "I cannot walk with these, for I have not tested them." So David took them off. Then he took his staff in his hand; and he chose for himself five smooth stones from the brook, and put them in a shepherd's bag, in a pouch which he had, and his sling was in his hand. And he drew near to the Philistine.* —1 SAMUEL 17:39-40

Here is a message I sent to the online Daniel Fast community in the spring of 2008:

As many of you know, I started another Daniel Fast this last Monday. It's a little different this time around. First, I am fasting for seven weeks instead of twenty-one days. Second, I am eating only three simple meals. Third, I am increasing my focus on God and His Word in such a way that I really do expect this to be one of the most significant spiritual experiences of my life.

You also may know that last year was a dark and difficult year for me, mainly because of being hit really hard financially. As a real estate investor serving the lower income population, I got caught in the middle of the real estate landslide and the subprime mortgage fall. Consequently, I had vacant houses, no buyers, a declining market, and many mortgage payments. I was all but wiped out!

God was so faithful . . . and brought me through. But I am now waging war on the lingering debt and pressing into God for a financial breakthrough.

Today in my quiet time I thought about David. The humble young shepherd had a giant to fight. One that seemed overpowering and had already proved to be a threat. I could identify with David's position. Our giants aren't exactly the same, but are still both very imposing!

In the verses above, we read about David taking off the armor that the soldiers had given him. Instead, he went to the brook and chose five smooth stones. We know the end of the story: David's weapon of choice and the five smooth stones were the death of Goliath, and David went on to be king of Israel!

I was moved to select five smooth stones of my own . . . and these I selected from the Living Water of Scripture. I went through my Bible and copied five verses into my journal. They all have to do with faith, God's provision, and my position with Christ.

These will be my weapons over this seven-week period. I will proclaim and memorize them. When I feel worry trying to enter my thinking, I will recite a verse and I will continue to fight the war with these five smooth stones from the Word of God.

Ephesians 6:12 tells us, "For we do not wrestle against flesh and blood, but against principalities, against powers, against the rulers of the darkness of this age, against spiritual hosts of wickedness in the heavenly places." It is in this realm where my five smooth stones are effective!

Coupling the power of God's Word with wise stewardship is what I believe will put me back on solid ground and into a level of faithful living that I will value forever.

Maybe you have a giant in your life, also. I encourage you to go to the Living Word of God and select your five smooth stones. Allow God to lift you up to victory and success!

The update to this story is that our amazing God is always faithful. I received hundreds of encouraging e-mails from my online friends, and the vast majority were reporting that they too would select their five smooth stones. For me, my Father showed me ways to create the income I would need, and He directed me to a bright future. The greatest prize is that my faith has developed and my confidence in the faithfulness and power of God is stronger than ever before. Amen! Our God is so good!

DAY 5

Take Every Thought Captive

For the weapons of our warfare are not carnal but mighty in God for pulling down strongholds, casting down arguments and every high thing that exalts itself against the knowledge of God, bringing every thought into captivity to the obedience of Christ.

—2 CORINTHIANS 10:4-5

Throughout the Daniel Fast, I hope you will become more aware of who you are and the makeup of your being:

You are a spirit.

You have a soul.

You live in a body.

In the passage above, we are reminded that our weapons and the war we fight are not of the flesh or in the physical world. Instead, they are of the Spirit and in the spiritual realm. The Word of God points us to the Kingdom of God—a reality that surrounds us and that is in us! It's a totally new way of thinking, different from the way our carnal, fleshly minds think.

So as we work to move our flesh and our minds toward Kingdom living, we must align every thought with the Word of God. Over and over again every day, we should ask ourselves, *What does God have to say about this?*

Every thought that is contrary to God's way must be "taken captive." Then we can toss that thought out and replace it with God's truth. His truth then becomes our activation point or our weapon.

- When a fearful thought comes into our minds, we take that lie, turn to the Word, find the promise, and then declare the truth.

- When the enemy tells us we're no good or defeated, we take that lie, turn to the Word, find the promise, and then declare the truth.

- When all the circumstances around us scream defeat and failure, we take that lie, turn to the Word, find the promise, and then declare the truth.

Taking every thought captive is a discipline. We must guard our hearts and minds. We must be alert to every notion that enters our thinking and measure it against God's Word, which wins the contest every time!

I once heard a pastor say, "Whenever you are confronted with a circumstance, you need to ask yourself three questions: What does God say about it? What does the enemy say about it? What are you going to say about it?"

I ask myself those questions all the time. It's a simple way to take every thought captive and choose Christ's way every time!

Joyce Meyer, a popular television teacher and bestselling author, wrote a book called *Battlefield of the Mind*. It's sold more than a million copies, and shows readers how to take thoughts captive and replace those that don't line up with the Word of God with those that do. The title says it clearly: the battle is in the mind, and it is important to guard the thoughts we allow to roll around in there. I like the way this popular prose puts it:

Watch your thoughts, for they become words.
Watch your words, for they become actions.
Watch your actions, for they become habits.
Watch your habits, for they become character.
Watch your character, for it becomes your destiny.

Our thoughts are important. So important that Paul gave us clear guidelines: "Finally, brethren, whatever things are true, whatever things are noble, whatever things are just, whatever things are pure, whatever things are lovely, whatever things are of good report, if there is any virtue and if there is anything praiseworthy—meditate on these things" (Philippians 4:8).

Your thoughts have power. Consider the things you are thinking about. Test them against the Word of God and then make the necessary changes. You will be amazed at the changes in your life as your thoughts become more like the thoughts of God.

DAY 6

The Kingdom of God

Jesus answered and said to him, "Most assuredly, I say to you, unless one is born again, he cannot see the kingdom of God."

—JOHN 3:3

The Kingdom of God is a separate place. It's an unseen reality that is under the jurisdiction of Jesus Christ the King. This Kingdom is open to all, but only accessible to those with the right credentials.

And what are those credentials? They are free and immediate when you believe in the Lord Jesus Christ and accept Him as your Savior. To cross into the Kingdom of God, you have to have identification that says, "This person belongs to Jesus Christ."

In John 3:3, Jesus explains that unless you are born again, you can't even see the Kingdom of God. But where is the Kingdom of God? Is it heaven? Do we have to wait until we pass from this world before we can see it?

Jesus answers these questions in Luke 17:20-21: "Now when He was asked by the Pharisees when the kingdom of God would come, He answered them and said, 'The kingdom of God does not come with observation; nor will they say, "See here!" or "See there!" For indeed, the kingdom of God is within you.'"

Jesus makes it clear that the Kingdom of God isn't a place to be seen with our natural eyes. It isn't a political system or reign on this earth. Rather, the Kingdom of God is a reality within us—a belief system or a way of thinking. It is different from the way the world thinks and can only be accessed through our faith in Christ and our willingness to operate our lives according to His ways.

When we shape our lives around God and His way of doing things, we live according to Kingdom principles and Kingdom laws. All those laws are clearly recorded in the Word of God, and it is by living by the Word that we have access to the good life and the power that God wants for us.

When Joshua was concerned about his ability to take over where Moses left off, God gave him simple instructions: "This Book of the Law shall not depart from your mouth, but you shall meditate in it day and night, that you may observe to do according to all that is written in it. For then you will make your way prosperous, and then you will have good success" (Joshua 1:8).

As a people consecrated under God, living a Spirit-led life, you and I are members of a different kingdom, the Kingdom of God. And we have different laws and standards by which we live. Those standards are available to us in God's Word!

The problem is that most members of the church have not changed their home addresses. Most are living by the world's standards and abiding by worldly laws rather than living by and realizing the amazing powers and promises Christ gained for us. It is sadly apparent in the body of Christ with rampant divorce, sickness, disease, promiscuity, financial pressures, and the like. But God says that power, victory, and freedom are all available to us.

When God told Joshua that following the law would make him prosperous and successful, it meant he would be moving forward in every area of his life. Joshua would achieve things when he put his trust in God and lived his life according to God's ways.

We have an even better offer because of Christ. We have Christ and His power living inside of us. But as long as those words remain just words on a page, they will have no effect. The truth of God's Word must become a reality for us—a reality that changes the way we think and believe. And then we can change the way we behave and the way we lead our lives.

Our citizenship in the Kingdom of God is waiting for us, but we must take the initiative. Not only must we want to live there, but we also must actually move there. Not physically, but in our hearts.

DAY 7

Please Lord, Take This Fear Away

Have I not commanded you? Be strong and of good courage; do not be afraid, nor be dismayed, for the LORD your God is with you wherever you go. —JOSHUA 1:9

Have you ever prayed and asked God to "take away this fear I feel" or perhaps "relieve me of this worry, Lord"? I prayed that prayer recently, and the Lord was quick to show me that He's already provided a way to free me from all worry, anxiety, and fear.

Joshua was afraid after Moses died, when he was handed the leadership over the Israelites. But God told him to be strong and of good courage. Then the Lord instructed him on how to achieve these character traits:

> *Only be strong and very courageous, that you may observe to do according to all the law which Moses My servant commanded you; do not turn from it to the right hand or to the left, that you may prosper wherever you go. This Book of the Law shall not depart from your mouth, but you shall meditate in it day and night, that you may observe to do according to all that is written in it. For then you will make your way prosperous, and then you will have good success.* —JOSHUA 1:7-8

The immediate response to feelings of fear, worry, or anxiety should be the Word of God. Instead of asking God to remove fear from us, we need to follow His instructions and fill our spirits and souls with the Word—the proven antidote for fear.

Pastor Bill Johnson wrote a book titled *Strengthen Yourself in the Lord* in which he shares how he overcomes doubt and moves into faith. He explains that he continues to pour the truth of God's Word into his spirit until the doubt gives way to faith. This may take time, but this is part of the good fight of faith. That's what we need to do with our souls. We must ask the Holy Spirit to control us, go to the living Word of God, and drink from it. If fear rises, we drink more. We keep drinking and feeding on the goodness of God until fear is gone and faith is strong.

God is not the author of fear; instead, the enemy uses it to paralyze our faith and make the Word of God of no effect. But we know the truth, and the truth sets us free from the bondages of fear. The truth is available for the taking, but we must take it.

The next time you hear yourself praying, "God, take this fear from me," do what the Lord told Joshua to do. Get into the Word. Meditate on it. Speak it out loud. Read it. Listen to it. Surround yourself with the purity of the Word of God, and soon the doubt and fear of the enemy will be washed away and only the truth will remain.

The process is rarely instantaneous, so we must keep on keeping on. "My brethren, count it all joy when you fall into various trials, knowing that the testing of your faith produces patience. But let patience have its perfect work, that you may be perfect and complete, lacking nothing" (James 1:2-4).

When we come up against doubt, our faith is being tested, but we can overcome doubt by patiently focusing on the promises of God until our faith becomes stronger. Then we will lack nothing! We merely need to follow the path the Lord has prepared for us.

DAY 8

Are You Politically Correct?

For our citizenship is in heaven, from which we also eagerly wait for the Savior, the Lord Jesus Christ. —PHILIPPIANS 3:20

We hear a lot about being "politically correct" these days. Much of it is good, and some is debatable. But today I am thinking about a different way to be politically correct.

Throughout the New Testament, followers of Jesus Christ are called to a different way of life: a higher calling that is separate from the world. First Peter 2:9 tells us, "But you are a chosen generation, a royal priesthood, a holy nation, His own special people, that you may proclaim the praises of Him who called you out of darkness into His marvelous light."

You and I are members of the Kingdom of God, and our politics are those of the almighty King Jesus: King of kings, Lord of lords, the Prince of Peace. The government of this Kingdom is on His shoulders.

When you think of the Kingdom of God with this political

structure, can you say that you are politically correct? Have you answered the call your Leader has for you? Do you recognize, know, and live by the spiritual laws of this Kingdom?

One lesson the Lord showed me in my meditations during the Daniel Fast is that while most of us proclaim Christ, we are not living as fully in Him as we can. Too much of the world distracts us from the glorious life we could have if we were sold out for the Kingdom of God. That doesn't mean we should be living in monasteries or communes. But it does call us to a life of faith that is different from what we have known before.

Jesus teaches that the Kingdom of God is within you (Luke 17:21). He also proclaims, "You are the light of the world. A city that is set on a hill cannot be hidden" (Matthew 5:14). He then goes on to say that our light should not be hidden, but available for all to see. In another parable Jesus teaches, "The kingdom of heaven is like a mustard seed, which a man took and sowed in his field, which indeed is the least of all the seeds; but when it is grown it is greater than the herbs and becomes a tree, so that the birds of the air come and nest in its branches" (Matthew 13:31-32).

That's you, me, and the church He's talking about. The Kingdom is within us. We should be so bright and so attractive that flocks of unbelievers are coming to us and nesting in our branches to hear the Good News of our King and His Kingdom!

The Bible says the Kingdom of God is a different place. And I have to ask if I truly consider myself a member of a "chosen generation, a royal priesthood, a holy nation, His own special people." Am I a citizen of an unseen but very real realm? Or do I feel more like an American or a Washingtonian? What nation do I consider to be my land, my home?

If I were politically correct in a Kingdom of God sense and a full-fledged member in the "holy nation," I would have total trust in my King, believing His every word and following His every lead. My heart would be full of peace, and I would make love my aim. I would believe more, worry less, and have complete confidence in my future no matter what condition the economy is in or if my circumstances look dark or threatening.

I want to be politically correct in the Kingdom to which I am called. I realize even as I write this message that my flesh needs more renewing and my spirit more training. What I know for sure is that I won't hear my King arguing on a campaign platform against His opponent, nor will I have to vote as to whether something really is or is not politically correct. In the holy nation, the King is always right, always fair, and always looking out for me. That's the nation I want for my life, my seed, and my seed's seed.

DAY 9

Why, Lord, Why?

Gideon said to Him, "O my lord, if the LORD is with us, why then has all this happened to us?" —JUDGES 6:13

Do you ever find yourself wondering about why you're going through such a rough time when God's promises are supposed to protect you? You've prayed, you've read your Bible, you attend church, you give your tithes . . . and yet the pressure doesn't seem to lift.

That's exactly what happened with Gideon. The Midianites were walking over the Israelites like they were a carpet! They stole their cattle, sheep, donkeys, and oxen. And just when the harvest was ready, the Midianites took over the land and let their camels eat the crops down to the stubble. The Bible says the camels were like locusts.

The Israelites were left impoverished and fled to caves and dens to hide from the invaders. Even Gideon was hiding in a pit when the angel of the Lord came to him.

The angel more or less said, "Why are you acting this way? Don't you know who you are? You are a child of the Most High God!"

That's when Gideon replied, "O my lord, if the LORD is with us, why then has all this happened to us?"

As the account continues, Gideon learns that because he hadn't recognized his position, he was allowing the enemy to steal and destroy what was rightfully his! He had the power of the Lord with him. In fact, God told him that because He would help him, defeating the Midianites would be like defeating one man.

Does any of this sound familiar to you? Do you ever feel like camels have eaten your harvest every month when you pay your bills? Do you feel like you are surrounded by enemies with all the pressures of this world coming in against you? Do you ever wish you could just go hide out in a cave to escape what seems like impending darkness all around?

Dear reader, too often we also forget who we are in Christ the King. We don't access the power that He won on the cross and then gave to us. Instead we stay in the pit and allow the enemy of this world to steal, kill, and destroy what is rightfully ours through the victory of Christ.

When Gideon realized his errors, he made sure everything was right before God and then prepared for battle, trusting in the Lord as his commander in chief. He did everything the Lord told him to do, which led him to victory over the invaders and caused the Israelites to receive all that had been stolen from them.

We can do the same thing! Read Judges 6 and 7 and see if you can find yourself in the Scriptures. Remember your identity in Christ and then access the same Lord that Gideon accessed. The victory is ours, but we need to take it.

So go identify your enemies, gird yourself in the weapons of our warfare, and fight your battles with your Commander in Chief in His rightful place. He only knows victory, and the victory is yours for the taking!

DAY 10

Set Your Mind for Good Things

For those who live according to the flesh set their minds on the things of the flesh, but those who live according to the Spirit, the things of the Spirit. —Romans 8:5

Do you ever have a bad day? You know the kind. You're giving it your all, but for some reason you just can't shake the worry you feel or the resentment that keeps sticking around.

The truth is, these are times when our flesh is reigning, and we need to pump up our spirit so it can take its rightful authority and position over our lives. I know that's a lot easier said than done, but I want to give you some practical tips to help you navigate through these stretching times.

First let me share a little personal testimony. The year 2007 was one of the most stretching of my entire life. I owned a real estate investment company, and due to the changes in the real estate market, I found myself without an income and owing thousands of dollars of monthly payments! There was no immediate solution. I had previously made a commitment to the Lord not to borrow any money and to work toward debt-free living.

At first, worry took over. I cried, pleaded, and begged God to help me. I don't think I have ever felt so desperate. But then I learned about living God's way, according to Kingdom principles. I really did experience a peace that passes all understanding. According to the world's standards I should have been climbing the walls with worry. But every time I felt worry and fear coming on, I turned my attention to the Lord. I prayed, read the Word, worshiped Him, and listened to Bible preachers or my audio Bible CDs. I did whatever I needed to do to get the worry out of my mind.

Instead of whining to my friends and family, I looked to the promises in God's Word and I did my best to keep my mind and

heart open to His leading. Over and over again, the Lord ministered to me. He kept telling me to hang on and trust Him.

I had been a Christian writer for many years but through various circumstances had gotten away from it and into real estate
investing. Well, it was clear that the Lord wanted me to get back
into writing because the doors in real estate were slamming shut
at record speed. Thankfully, I had learned that in times of trouble
I need to find refuge in the secret place of the Most High. I ran
to the Lord and took refuge in Him. And then He started giving
me writing assignments; He started showing me things to write
about.

The journey was definitely a fight for faith. This is walking in
faith—living and acting according to the Word of God. It was not
always an easy walk, but it has been fulfilling, and the rewards are
superior to anything I've ever known.

One thing I know for sure: God only has victory in mind for
us. He always has a sure way out of any trouble, just like Jesus
said: "These things I have spoken to you, that in Me you may have
peace. In the world you will have tribulation; but be of good cheer,
I have overcome the world" (John 16:33).

So what do we do to be "in Him"? We study His Word and
meditate on it so it becomes our truth. Not just a good philosophy
or a part of religion. The truth must come off those pages and enter
our hearts where it can flourish and bring us the peace and fulfill-
ment our Father wants us to have. When we surrender our thinking to God's thinking, then we are truly free!

Jesus is saying to you, "If you abide in My word, you are My
disciples indeed. And you shall know the truth, and the truth shall
make you free" (John 8:31-32).

To abide is to live or dwell. Jesus wants us to live in Him through
His Word. He wants us to choose a Spirit-led life over a flesh-led
existence. He is the Way, the Truth, and the Life!

DAY 11

Living Water

If anyone thirsts, let him come to Me and drink. He who believes in Me, as the Scripture has said, out of his heart will flow rivers of living water. —JOHN 7:37-38

Water is a primary element in the Daniel Fast. It is the only beverage we consume. Even when we aren't fasting, the human body depends on safe water for life. In fact, just before I started writing this devotion I realized I had neglected a basil plant I was growing. The poor little thing was so wilted that the leaves were starting to dry up. I thought for sure I had lost it, but I decided to water it anyway. Within the hour, the little trooper was perky, green, and full of life. It was the water!

In this passage, Jesus teaches us about a different kind of water—living water from the Holy Spirit. He tells us to come to Him and drink when we are thirsty.

As a seasoned woman (that's code for saying I am definitely in the second half of my life) and a maturing Christian, I have learned a powerful lesson about turning to Jesus to drink from His living water. It actually was Dr. Phil McGraw, the well-known American television personality, talk-show host, and former psychologist, who helped me learn this valuable principle. Let me explain.

Dr. Phil teaches married couples that when they are going through hard times, they should not turn away from each other or go outside the marriage for comfort or solutions. Rather, they should turn toward each other and work out their problems together.

This advice resonated in my soul when I felt so burdened by life's pressures that I could almost feel my knees buckle. Instead of turning to the world for solutions or getting stuck in fear and doubt, I turned to my High Priest. I cried out to Him and asked for His advice, His comfort, and His peace.

Oh, our Lord is so faithful. He hears our cries and comforts us. He ministered to me in dynamic and life-giving ways through His Word, Christian teachers, prayer, Scripture meditation, and friends. He led me out of the dark place and showed me solutions I never would have thought of on my own.

I drank from the living water Jesus serves so generously. And then as I was restored, I was able to offer living water to others, just as He said, "Out of his [her] heart will flow rivers of living water."

Since that experience, I have set my mind on drinking a lot of living water from the Word of God, and bit by bit, I find myself changed into a strong and able woman of God. I liken this process to a tall glass filled with dark, murky water with a pitcher of water on either side. One pitcher is filled with more murky water from the world. The other pitcher is filled with clear living water from the Word of God.

If I empty the glass and refill it with the water of the world, it will be as murky as before. But if I empty the glass and fill it with the living water from the Word of God, the water in the glass will be good enough to drink and to offer to others.

As you proceed through the Daniel Fast, consider the source of the water you pour into your heart. Is it the living water of Jesus or the contaminated water from the world? Choose life! Choose the living water. It is safe, sweet, and it truly quenches your thirst. And once you are full, the living water will overflow from your life so that you can help quench the thirst of others. Amen!

DAY 12

Set Your Mind on Things Above

If then you were raised with Christ, seek those things which are above, where Christ is, sitting at the right hand of God. Set your mind on things above, not on things on the earth.

—Colossians 3:1-2

Not long ago, I received a question from a woman on the Daniel Fast. She asked me how much is okay to eat for a snack while fasting. I encouraged her to make a decision about how much is okay for a snack *before* snack time comes. For example, if you decide that twelve almonds is a nice snack for the afternoon, stick with that amount.

This reminded me of Colossians 3:2 that says to "set your mind on things above," and the tremendous tool this discipline gives us. Setting our minds is making a decision, and once the decision is made, sticking with it—just like when we're fasting. We make a decision about what foods are okay to eat and which are not, and then during the fast we stick to our decision.

There are so many things that we can make conscious decisions about that would save us so much pain and anguish. For example, many years ago I made a decision to not gossip. I set my mind to never talk negatively about a person or to pass on private information. While I admit I have not been 100 percent perfect in that area, I am pretty close. And in the few times that I've blundered, I was conscious of it right away and could repent (change), ask for forgiveness, and move on with a greater resolve.

In fact, I had lunch a couple of weeks ago with a business associate and valued friend named Steve. He is what I like to call a "pre-Christian." I had not seen Steve for a few years, so we had a lot of catching up to do. He asked me about a situation in which someone had really done me wrong. I had the opportunity to blast on the person, but I chose not to. Instead I made a couple of neutral comments about him and his situation. Then Steve paid me a treasured compliment, "You know, I've known you a long time, and in all those years I have never heard you say a bad thing about anyone."

Wow! I have to admit Steve's words blessed me. He picked up on a part of my behavior in which my natural self was conformed to Christ living in me: my decision to not gossip. I had set my mind on things above, and it served as a positive witness to Steve.

There are other areas in our lives where we need to "set our minds on things above" or on the commands of the Lord. For example, throughout Scripture we read that we should never come before the Lord empty-handed. I was struck by that command just last week, realizing there are many times when I come to church with nothing to give. I am a cheerful tither and generally give my monthly tithe at the beginning of each month. But many times during the rest of the month, I don't give anything.

But the Lord impressed on me that I should never come before Him empty-handed. I made a decision to follow that command. Now I will always leave my house with something to give to the Lord. Sometimes it's a batch of homemade cookies for the church coffee hour. Occasionally I bring some gifts for the children's ministry or donate some books for the prison ministry. And then there are the financial gifts for outreaches our body is doing.

Another area where I set my mind was to "owe no one anything except to love" him or her. In the fall of 2007 I made a decision to not borrow any more money for anything and to get out of debt as soon as possible. Deuteronomy 28:12 says, "You shall lend to many nations, but you shall not borrow." So I plan to live a debt-free life. I made a contract with myself to never borrow again. This was a quality decision that I will continue to follow so I can proclaim, "Owe no one anything except to love one another, for he who loves another has fulfilled the law" (Romans 13:8).

These examples just scratch the surface of how we can "set our minds on things above." The point is this: if we want to be conformed to the ways of God and the image of Christ, then we need to make these kinds of conscious decisions and stick to them. We need to make them *before* the need for the decision comes about.

We can decide to not overspend, overeat, or overplay. As followers of Christ we can decide not to look at pornography, not to develop unhealthy relationships with coworkers, and not to flirt with things that can bring us or others harm. We can decide to attend church every Sunday, share with the poor, and meet with the Lord every day for an intimate time of prayer.

We are called to set our minds on things above. What does that mean for you and your life? Is the Holy Spirit nudging you to take a stand in an area and make a quality decision to change . . . and then stick with it?

Take a few minutes even right now and listen to the Lord. Ask Him if there are areas of your life where you need to set your mind on things above, and then lift the commitment to the Lord, ask the Holy Spirit to guide and direct you, and stick to it. You will be blessed!

DAY 13

I Know the Plans I Have for You

"For I know the plans I have for you," declares the LORD, "plans to prosper you and not to harm you, plans to give you hope and a future." —JEREMIAH 29:11, NIV

This is one of my favorite verses. It's so encouraging and full of promise. Wow! The Lord has plans for me to prosper and have a good future. That's good news.

So how do we discover the plans our Father and Creator has just for us? Do we wait for the writing to appear on the wall or for a messenger to arrive at our door? As inviting as that sounds, I don't think that's the answer. We tap into God's best for us when we start dreaming and planning while staying sensitive to His voice.

Getting quiet before the Lord, submitting yourself to Him, and seeking the Holy Spirit's help is a powerful experience. Ask the Holy Spirit to work through you and reveal the Father's plans for you.

Establishing short- and long-term goals will boost your success and lead you toward those dreams and accomplishments that the Lord plants in your heart. For every good work He calls you to do, your Father will provide the tools to succeed. But you need to search your heart and discover what may be forgotten hopes and dreams . . . and then develop goals to reach them.

Most people have never learned to tap into their dreams or how to set goals for their lives. Instead, they go aimlessly on life's journey and figure things out along the way. Sadly, this approach can lead to a life of mediocrity and disappointment. But we can choose a different approach.

Planning and writing goals is a proven system for success. And just think how successful we could be if our goals and plans were undergirded, protected, and fortified by the Lord! So why don't we plan and write goals? Why don't we invest the time, energy, and meditation necessary to discover the plans the Lord has for us?

I think the answer is no different for Christians than it is for non-Christians. Many people don't think goals are important. And if people don't value planning and goal setting, they don't do it. Many people don't know how to set goals or how to create plans to fulfill them; still others fear rejection or failure.

Throughout the Bible, God shows by example that He is one for planning, details, and success. He planned the creation of the universe to take six days. He planned in minute detail how the Tabernacle would be constructed. He counts the hairs on our heads and the number of our days.

He also likes things to be in writing: the Ten Commandments, the Word of God, and the plans He told Habakkuk to write, just to name a few. And Jeremiah 29:11 says that He has plans for you! But before those plans can move into action, we must do our part.

I love the line, "You will never rise above the vision you have for yourself." There is great truth in that adage. What is the vision you have for yourself? What do you know of the plans your Father has for you? What do you see in your future? These are all questions we can answer as we set goals and develop plans for our lives, realizing that the Lord wants us to have goodness and success.

So what will it take for us to dream dreams, make plans, and write goals? It seems that it comes down to wanting the future that God has in His mind for us and then deciding to take action.

You've heard the line, "Today is the first day of the rest of your life." You have the rest of your life before you, and you can begin today to start thinking about and making plans for your future. What do you want for your family? your career? your faith? your health?

Let's not allow the obstacles that keep the masses down to also keep us from realizing all God wants for us. Let's make a quality decision to be quiet before the Lord, to listen to Him, to imagine our desires, to make plans, and to write them down.

DAY 14

Lose the Shackles

> *Then Caleb quieted the people before Moses, and said, "Let us go up at once and take possession, for we are well able to overcome it."* —NUMBERS 13:30

Do you remember the story about the twelve spies that God instructed Moses to send into the Promised Land? God brought the Israelites out of Egypt and freed them from slavery in a miraculous way by parting the Red Sea. While in their transitional place, He fed them with bread from heaven. He gave them quail to eat. He set up structures and systems for their existence. Still the Israelites complained and grumbled. Finally, after traveling for two years, they drew near to the Promised Land.

The Lord had already given them the land, but they needed to apprehend it before they could possess it. So the spies went into Canaan for forty days so they could see what they were in for. Ten of the spies came back with a bad report: while the land was fertile, abundant, and rich with milk and honey, the obstacles were too big. The men in the land were large and fierce and too much for the bedraggled Israelites to overcome.

Only Caleb and Joshua saw things differently. They, too, saw the land of milk and honey, and they also saw the imposing forces that would come against them. But they believed God and trusted Him to help them take the land that He had promised. They took God at His word.

Whom did the masses believe? What picture did they accept as their vision for the future? The slave-minded Israelites were accustomed to hardship. That was their comfort zone. Even when God blessed them with good things, they still grumbled. Even though they were out of Egypt, the Egyptian mind-set was not out of them.

So they accepted the bad report as the truth, and they wandered in the desert for the rest of their lives.

We know the end of the story—the real truth: God gave the new generation of thinkers and leaders all the help they needed to take what He had already given them through His promise. What did they need for their weapons? Faith—faith in God and trust that He would do what He said He would do.

We look at the poor wandering Israelites and imagine that we would be different. *Surely if I were alive then I would be like Caleb and Joshua and trust in the Lord,* we think to ourselves. But is that really true? Are we not shackled by beliefs that are just as paralyzing and just as damaging?

How many of us are chained to beliefs of inadequacy, guilt, or shame that result in a poverty mentality that keeps us wandering in the same old land we've been in forever? How many of us are following the actions of our ancestors that keep us bound in traditions disguised as truth? How many of us are weighed down with fear and anxiety so we don't take risks to trust in an unseen God who decrees lofty promises?

Right now, no matter where you are in life, you have an opportunity to be like the ten pessimists and the millions of men and women who believed them. Or you can be like the few people who stepped out in faith and realized all God wanted to give them. The choice is ours: we can leave God's promises unrealized or we can gain the victory!

Remember God's call to us in Deuteronomy 30:19: "I call heaven and earth as witnesses today against you, that I have set before you life and death, blessing and cursing; therefore choose life, that both you and your descendants may live."

Let's step out in faith and chose life!

DAY 15

Be Rooted and Built Up in Christ

> *As you therefore have received Christ Jesus the Lord, so walk in Him, rooted and built up in Him and established in the faith, as you have been taught, abounding in it with thanksgiving.*
>
> —COLOSSIANS 2:6-7

I think we all can agree, these are turbulent times we're living in. Whether we look at the economy, the crime rate, societal issues, politics, world affairs, or the pressures we face day to day, by the world's standards these are very shaky, unstable days.

That's why, even though it was written two thousand years ago, this word from the apostle Paul is so right-on for us today. To find our stability, we must be rooted and established in Christ and His ways. And when we come up against pressures, concerns, or trials, He is there to build us up and keep us strong.

How do we get rooted and built up in Christ? It's by bringing Him into the number one position in every part of our lives. That includes our marriages, parenting, friendships, careers, work, finances, entertainment, volunteerism, study, and plans for our future.

Jesus told us that He is always with us, which is extremely comforting. The writer of Hebrews also says, "Marriage is honorable among all, and the bed undefiled; but fornicators and adulterers God will judge. Let your conduct be without covetousness; be content with such things as you have. For He Himself has said, 'I will never leave you nor forsake you'" (Hebrews 13:4-5).

The presence of Jesus inside of us and with us is promised. So "Lord, what do You have to say about this?" can be constantly on our tongues. Seeking God's wisdom in His Word can be a normal practice for us. And when we still don't know what to do, we can get godly counsel from a pastor or friends who are mature in Christ.

Being rooted means going deep! It means investing the time and energy into getting to know God and His ways and devoting time to be with Him so we can have an intimate relationship with Him. And the deeper those roots dig down, the more stable we will be. We won't be knocked off center when storms enter our lives. We will know what to do and where to go.

We can see this type of living unfold in James 1:2-8:

Count it all joy when you fall into various trials, knowing that the testing of your faith produces patience. But let patience have its perfect work, that you may be perfect and complete, lacking nothing. If any of you lacks wisdom, let him ask of God, who gives to all liberally and without reproach, and it will be given to him. But let him ask in faith, with no doubting, for he who doubts is like a wave of the sea driven and tossed by the wind. For let not that man suppose that he will receive anything from the Lord; he is a double-minded man, unstable in all his ways.

We can become stable in all our ways, firm in faith, and confident in the ways of God. Take a few minutes and ask yourself these questions:

- How can I become more rooted in Christ?
- What are three things I can do to increase my knowledge of Him and His ways?
- What time am I willing to set aside for the sole (or soul) purpose of studying the Word of God so that I can become firmly established in His truth?

Make plans to grow in Christ so that when times of trouble come, you will be ready! Our Lord beckons us to "come." He calls, but we must respond. Can you hear Him calling you now?

DAY 16

Not by Bread Alone

Now when the tempter came to Him, he said, "If You are the Son of God, command that these stones become bread." But He answered and said, "It is written, 'Man shall not live by bread alone, but by every word that proceeds from the mouth of God.'"

—MATTHEW 4:3-4

Wow! You are now more than two weeks into your Daniel Fast. You are likely past the big hunger pangs and cravings. But leavened bread is still out of your diet, so perhaps this passage of Scripture is even more meaningful to you than when you were able to bite into crusty French bread or a morning bagel.

One of the benefits of the Daniel Fast is that we become more aware of what we are eating. Hopefully this awareness will create habits that will improve your health for months and years to come.

We can also become more aware of what we feed our spirits and our souls. Are they well nourished? Are we feeding them wholesome food and not contaminated goods?

Jesus teaches us that we don't live only by physical bread, but instead—and even more important—the spiritual food found in God's Word. Just as our physical bodies need to be nourished each and every day, so do our spirits.

The mainstay of that nutrition is the Bible, then we can have what I call "side dishes" from Christian books, sermons, Bible studies, and Christian television. But we need to make sure we have time every day in God's holy Word so He can speak to us and minister to us.

Likewise, we need to make sure we are feeding our souls a healthy diet that brings life and not death. Our Father tells us that we have a choice between life and death, and He tells us to choose life. That includes the kind of information that enters our minds through people, the media, the Internet, television, books, conversations, and other influences we encounter.

Do you have some inputs in your life that may not be giving you the best food for your soul? Are the programs you watch on television healthy and pure? Or are they contaminated and laced with toxic information? How about the Internet? The radio? The books you read? Or the conversations you have with friends?

Just as we need to guard our bodies and make wise choices about what we eat, we must also guard our eyes and our ears as to what is allowed to enter our souls. And we must guard our mouths as to what words we say.

The more you feed your spirit with the Word of God, the better you will find that you care for your soul and your body. Make sure your spirit is well fed, and then carefully choose the food you present to your soul and your body. That's the way to health in all areas of your life.

DAY 17

It Wasn't about the Money!

And again I say to you, it is easier for a camel to go through the eye of a needle than for a rich man to enter the kingdom of God.
—MATTHEW 19:24

This is a verse that seems to trip up a lot of Christians, and it certainly fuels the argument that to be a good follower of Christ one should be poor or at best middle class.

Jesus' reference to the "eye of a needle" was likely a gate in the wall surrounding the city of Jerusalem called "Needle's Eye." It was so low that a camel would have to be unloaded of all that it carried and then get down on its knees to get through to the other side. The passage was very small, and it took a great deal of coaxing for the owner to get his camel to come through.

Basically, Jesus is saying that it's nearly impossible for a rich man to enter the Kingdom of God. But it isn't the money that keeps a rich man from entering; it is where the rich man places his dependence. Jesus is saying that people with money often rely on their wealth to solve all their problems. They don't sense a need for God or His way of living. Thus the teaching in 1 Timothy 6:10: "For the love of money is a root of all kinds of evil." It's not the money. It's the love, trust, and dependence on money that is evil and makes it so difficult for people to enter into the Kingdom of God.

We see the same thing today. People are so focused on making and spending money that they don't even consider God. Their self-worth isn't measured by their character or their relationship with the Father, but rather their position, their possessions, and the people they know.

The priorities of the world are easily observed by just flipping through a magazine, clicking on Yahoo pages, or switching the television channel. The absence of God is very apparent, and the love of money is manifested in an explosive way.

Sadly, these values seem to be alive and thriving in the church as well. Too often we look to the world's system for directions in living. Consequently, God's plan for our lives goes untapped and unmet. I have to admit that I was like that for many years in my Christian life. It wasn't until I had the invisible crutches of my middle-class life knocked out from under me that I turned to God as my Provider and began learning what Kingdom living really is all about.

I am so thankful for what I know now. For me it took becoming financially desperate to realize that I was depending on money and the world's system for my livelihood. Thank God I now live in the Kingdom of God. I finally got it! And the great news is that my Father has opened the heavens of His resources and is pouring them down on me.

Am I specially chosen by God to receive His blessings? Yes! We all are chosen, but we also have to choose right back. God gives us the choice whether we will enter His Kingdom. It's our choice whether we will align ourselves with His ways. And the way is not difficult. We can examine our hearts and present them to the Holy Spirit, who will show us where we need to change. We can make Christ the Lord over every part of our lives, including our finances.

Open your heart to the Lord today in the area of your finances. Is the Lord the Overseer and Source of your funds? Is He your Provider? Examine yourself and ask the Holy Spirit to help you draw even closer to the Lord by submitting this area of your life to Him so that you can fully partake of the Kingdom of God. It truly is the good life.

DAY 18

Who Do You Say That I Am?

When Jesus came into the region of Caesarea Philippi, He asked His disciples, saying, "Who do men say that I, the Son of Man, am?"

So they said, "Some say John the Baptist, some Elijah, and others Jeremiah or one of the prophets."

He said to them, "But who do you say that I am?"

—Matthew 16:13-15

The passage above is a familiar one. Simon Bar-Jonah's response to the question garnered him his new name from Jesus: Peter, which means *rock*.

As I read that passage today, the Holy Spirit prompted me to ask this same question of you and of me: "Who do you say that I am?"

This isn't a question for our minds or our intellects or even our traditional beliefs. Today this question is directed to our hearts: "Who do you say that I am?"

Is Jesus a far-off figure that is part of our religious tradition? The one we celebrate on Christmas and Easter? Is He the painting on the Sunday school classroom wall? Or is He the Savior we read about in the Bible and look forward to meeting one day?

Today He is asking us, "Who do you say that I am?"

For many years, Jesus was a far-off figure for me. I knew a lot *about* Him. I even taught many others about Him. I wrote inspirational pieces about Him. And I said many prayers to Him. But it wasn't until I got desperate for Jesus to be more in my life that I actually started *knowing* Him.

This knowing didn't come overnight. Instead, there was a period of deep and steadfast seeking that put my spirit in closer communion with His. Jesus wasn't hiding from me. Instead, I didn't know how to find Him in the intimate way that He wanted to befriend me. Even now, I am not as "tight" with Him as I know I can be, but every day I draw closer and closer.

What I know to be true is what the Scripture teaches us in James 4:8: "Draw near to God and He will draw near to you." Until we make the decision to get to know our Lord by setting aside the time and quieting ourselves on a consistent basis, the relationship we want won't happen.

That's why the question, "Who do you say that I am?" is so poignant. Is Jesus a priority in our lives, or do we wait until we have time? Is He a person with whom we can have an intimate and caring relationship? Or is He someone who lived a long time ago and we will wait to see Him in heaven?

Over the past several years, my relationship with Christ has grown from an ethereal concept to a deep and abiding relationship. He is who I go to for all my needs. He's the first one I greet in the morning and the one I talk to throughout the day. Many times He talks to me, and I can hear His voice and know what He's saying, since I've developed the "ears to hear."

I am so grateful that I have moved from knowing *about* Jesus to really knowing Him. I hope you will take the opportunity over the next several days to answer the question Jesus asks you: "Who do you say that I am?"

DAY 19

Going Deeper with the Word of God

Trust in the LORD with all your heart, and lean not on your own understanding; in all your ways acknowledge Him, and He shall direct your paths. —PROVERBS 3:5-6

During one of my morning times with God, I was thinking about trust, which led me to one of my favorite places in the Old Testament: Proverbs 3:5-6. I looked at the verses, let them roll around in my head for a while, and then started mining the truths in this short yet powerful passage.

First I looked up "trust." The Hebrew word is *chasah*, which means "to hope in; to make our refuge." The definition reminded me of Psalm 91:1-2, which says, "He who dwells in the secret place of the Most High shall abide under the shadow of the Almighty. I will say of the LORD, 'He is my refuge and my fortress; my God, in Him I will trust.'"

Then I looked up "heart." The Hebrew word is *leb*, which means a person's intellect, personality, emotions, spirit, and innermost self. Our "heart" is who we are; it is what is tested and searched out by God. The heart and spirit are often used interchangeably. It is that innermost part of us that is born-again when we accept Christ as the Lord of our lives. Jesus also told us, "You shall love the LORD your God with all your heart, with all your soul, and with all your mind" (Matthew 22:37).

The next word I searched out was "ways." The Hebrew word is *derek*. It means a road, a course, or a mode of action.

And finally I looked up "acknowledge," which is *yada'* in Hebrew. This means intimate exchanges; for marriage it means intercourse where new life is conceived and birthed. With the Lord it is intimate time in prayer and meditation that reveals His truth and births blessings and victories in our lives.

So when I put it all together, this is what I heard this Scripture saying to me: make the Lord my refuge and my secret place for every part of me. That means the way I think, the way I feel, the way I behave, the way I approach life. I am to set aside my own thinking, which has been trained by the world and is so deficient when compared with the almighty God. In everything I do, big or small, I need to seek the Lord by coming to Him in prayer and meditating on His Word. Then He *will* direct every step I take. He will move heaven and earth to make my way successful.

What an opportunity the Lord gives us if we follow His way of doing things. Not our way, but His way. That is walking in the Spirit. That is living by faith.

So what must we do to tap into the powerhouse God offers? Basically we must lose ourselves and seek God. Simple? Yes! But it takes a firm decision and a quality commitment to do it. Choosing God is not a shallow option. And it doesn't happen overnight. If you were to interview the men and women who have dynamic relationships with God, you would quickly learn that they bury themselves in the Word of God on a consistent basis. They have developed habits of prayer, meditation, Bible study, and learning about our Lord. They have made knowing God and renewing their minds with the truth of His Word their primary goal. And from the knowledge they gain from the intimate relationship they have with their Father, they live their lives.

Every person has the same opportunity to trust in the Lord with all of his or her heart. We can be renewed. We can be led by God. We can have a blessed and powerful life. But it takes an unceasing commitment.

Is it worth it? Well, let's see. Do I want my way or God's way? Hmmm . . . no contest! That's why I do whatever I need to do to trust in the Lord with all my heart, lean not on my own understanding, and in all my ways acknowledge Him so He can direct my paths.

That's a powerful way to live. I am my own testimony! Like the blind man in John 9:25 (NIV) who said, "I was blind but now I see," my life has been forever changed because of the wondrous works of God. I know the before, and I am living in the after. He didn't bless me because I was so good or so special or so smart. No, God has made amazing differences in my life because He loves me. He wants to bless me. I am His precious child. For me, this is the best way to live, by far. The peace, joy, and love are so valuable that I would have it no other way!

The amazing truth is that anyone can have the same blessings. The opportunity is right there for anyone willing to follow the ways of the Lord.

DAY 20

If Jesus Is the Firstborn, What Does That Say about You?

He is the image of the invisible God, the firstborn over all creation. —Colossians 1:15

Have you ever heard a biblical truth and found yourself almost awestruck? That's what happened to me when I meditated on this Scripture and the thought that Jesus is the firstborn. In Romans 8:29, He is called "the firstborn among many brethren."

Firstborn means exactly what the word says: the first or eldest child of a family. The Greek word is *prototokos*, which means the first to be born or the eldest child. The position is not that of stature, but rather of chronological order: first.

So if Jesus is the firstborn among many brethren, what does that say about you and me? What happens when we couple this truth with that of Romans 2:11, "For there is no partiality with God." Or Romans 8:15, which says, "For you did not receive the spirit of bondage again to fear, but you received the Spirit of adoption by whom we cry out, 'Abba, Father.'"

I asked myself the question that brought shivers to my soul: if Jesus is the firstborn, then what does that say about me?

I encourage you to ask yourself the same question. The answer is amazing. But we won't get the full impact of this truth unless we take it in and let it roll around in our minds and hearts until it transforms our thoughts and our identities. Do you really see yourself as a younger sibling to Jesus? He is the Son of God. You are a child of God also. You are a joint heir with Christ. Not because I said it or because of a denominational perspective. You are a child of God and a joint heir with Christ because God says so!

We are not lowly urchins. Romans 8:16-17 tells us who we are: "The Spirit Himself bears witness with our spirit that we are children of God, and if children, then heirs—heirs of God and joint heirs with Christ, if indeed we suffer with Him, that we may also be glorified together."

You and I are joint heirs with Christ!

Another very interesting element in this mix is something few Christians consider. When God sent Jesus, He was His only begotten Son. But when Jesus rose from the dead and ascended to heaven, He was the firstborn. The only Son becomes the firstborn because of the Cross. No longer is Jesus the *only* Son. Jesus made it possible for you and me to join the family. Do you realize the truth and reality in all of this? The Son of God became the Son of Man so the sons of men could become the sons of God.

As born-again women and men, we are bona fide members of the family of God. Jesus was first and made it possible for us to have all the same rights, privileges, and benefits. I hope you will take a few minutes and ponder what this truth means to you—let it sink in—ask yourself the question, "If Jesus is the firstborn, then what does that say about me?" Then the next time you feel lowly and hopeless, remember who you are: you are a loved, cherished, esteemed joint heir with Jesus, the firstborn of all creation!

Be blessed in your identity!

DAY 21

Do You Still Feel Like You're in the Fire?

And these three men, Shadrach, Meshach, and Abed-Nego, fell down bound into the midst of the burning fiery furnace. Then King Nebuchadnezzar was astonished; and he rose in haste and spoke, saying to his counselors, "Did we not cast three men bound into the midst of the fire?"

They answered and said to the king, "True, O king."

*"Look!" he answered, "I see four men loose, walking in the midst of the fire; and they are not hurt, and the form of the fourth is like the Son of God." —*DANIEL 3:23-25

Of course, the amazing fact of this story is that three men went into the fiery furnace, but four men were seen walking around amidst the flames. Long before being thrown into the furnace, the Hebrew men had faith in their God and His promises. "Be strong and of good courage, do not fear nor be afraid of them; for the LORD your God, He is the One who goes with you. He will not leave you nor forsake you" (Deuteronomy 31:6). And here in the midst of this death chamber was the presence of God watching over and protecting His children. Scholars call the fourth man in the furnace a Christophany, which is a preincarnate appearance of Jesus, the Messiah. God's faithfulness showed up.

But let's look at some of the other details. One is that the men were bound. They could do nothing on their own. There are times in our lives when we are so bound by the troubles in this world that we can do nothing in our own strength. Sometimes the restraints are brought on by others and not our own doing—as in the case of the Hebrew men. But whether those things that bind us are self-inflicted because of bad choices we've made or are caused by the sins of others, the answer is always the same: trust in the Lord. That's what these men did. Nebuchadnezzar saw and exclaimed, "I see four men loose!" The restraints were gone! Even before they were out of the fire, they were free, and the Lord was there standing by them.

The same should be true for us. Even if you've faithfully fasted for three weeks, you still may be in the midst of fiery circumstances. But even though you haven't realized the victory with your eyes, you are free.

If we have faith in the victory, it is already ours. Jesus said in Mark 11:24: "Therefore I say to you, whatever things you ask when you pray, believe that you receive them, and you will have them."

Shadrach, Meshach, and Abed-Nego had already received what was theirs. They weren't out of the fire yet. But they were free to walk around in a furnace that was seven times hotter than it usually was—a heat so high that it killed the executioners.

There may be times when the challenges of this world seem

almost unbearable for those who don't know Christ. But God promises that He will always care for His children: "No temptation has overtaken you except such as is common to man; but God is faithful, who will not allow you to be tempted beyond what you are able, but with the temptation will also make the way of escape, that you may be able to bear it" (1 Corinthians 10:13).

In the book of Daniel, the men who depended on pagan gods were killed, yet the men who depended on Almighty God were able to escape as their Lord provided a way in the midst of evil circumstances. Nebuchadnezzar was astonished by this powerful God; he simply couldn't believe what he was seeing:

> *Nebuchadnezzar went near the mouth of the burning fiery furnace and spoke, saying, "Shadrach, Meshach, and Abed-Nego, servants of the Most High God, come out, and come here." Then Shadrach, Meshach, and Abed-Nego came from the midst of the fire. And the satraps, administrators, governors, and the king's counselors gathered together, and they saw these men on whose bodies the fire had no power; the hair of their head was not singed nor were their garments affected, and the smell of fire was not on them.*
>
> *Nebuchadnezzar spoke, saying, "Blessed be the God of Shadrach, Meshach, and Abed-Nego, who sent His Angel and delivered His servants who trusted in Him, and they have frustrated the king's word, and yielded their bodies, that they should not serve nor worship any god except their own God! Therefore I make a decree that any people, nation, or language which speaks anything amiss against the God of Shadrach, Meshach, and Abed-Nego shall be cut in pieces, and their houses shall be made an ash heap; because there is no other God who can deliver like this."*
>
> *Then the king promoted Shadrach, Meshach, and Abed-Nego in the province of Babylon.* —DANIEL 3:26-30

Nebuchadnezzar was impressed, but not converted. He saw the power of God through his natural eyes, and he recognized God as being better than all other gods. This kind of mental assent is rampant in the world today. Many people believe there is a god. Of these, some believe the God of the Bible is the only true God, and of these, many even believe in Christ. But mental assent is not conversion, and this is where a lot of people miss it.

My prayer for you is that this Daniel Fast has ushered you into a more real and meaningful relationship with your Father so that you will never "miss out" again. I hope you have received answers to your prayers and insights about how you can partner with Christ as you feed your soul, strengthen your spirit, and renew your body. And I pray that when you look back over these past weeks you are encouraged to see how your loving Father has worked in your life.

Amen!

Frequently Asked Questions

Q. *Our whole family is going to go on the Daniel Fast. Do think this is a healthy eating plan for children? My oldest is six years old.*

A. According to Jewish law, children are not responsible for their actions until they reach "the age of majority," generally thirteen years for boys and twelve for girls. At this time, children start to bear their own responsibility for Jewish ritual law, tradition, and ethics and are privileged to participate in all areas of Jewish community life. Prior to this, the child's parents hold the responsibility for the child's adherence to Jewish law and tradition. Health and growth issues also must be considered for preteen children. The main thing you want to teach your children about fasting is the fact that it's part of our spiritual discipline. I think you will be most effective with your children if you ask them which foods they would like to restrict so they can experience the impact of the fast.

Q. *How long should I fast? Is the Daniel Fast always twenty-one days?*

A. The Daniel Fast is usually done for twenty-one days; however, that is not a required time period. I have used the fast for as few as ten days and for as many as fifty. Consider your purpose for fasting, then ask the Holy Spirit to show you how long you should fast. Even as I write this answer, I plan to fast at least twenty-one days, but I will "check in" with the Holy Spirit as the time draws to a close to see if I should fast longer. Individual situations can help determine the length of the fast.

Q. *I didn't see _____ on the food list. Can I eat it on the Daniel Fast?*

A. One of the easiest ways to determine whether a food is okay for the Daniel Fast is to think of it as a vegan diet with even more restrictions. Therefore, all fruits and vegetables are allowed; all whole grains, seeds, and nuts are allowed; and all good quality oils, herbs, and spices are allowed. Animal products are restricted; all sweeteners are restricted; all chemicals and man-made products are restricted; and all alcohol, caffeine, and other stimulants are restricted.

Q. *Is it okay to have sex with my spouse during the Daniel Fast?*

A. Paul teaches about abstaining from marital relations in 1 Corinthians 7:5: "Do not deprive one another except with consent for a time, that you may give yourselves to fasting and prayer; and come together again so that Satan does not tempt you because of your lack of self-control." While married couples are not required to abstain from marital relations during their fast, many find it a powerful experience as they bring greater focus on the Lord and also find other ways to express love and respect to one another.

Q. *Why can't we have herbal tea? It's a plant with no chemicals or sweeteners.*

A. This is a very common question. The reason there is no tea on the Daniel Fast is because in Daniel 1:12 we read that the prophet requested only "water to drink." Therefore, the only beverage on the Daniel Fast is water. You can embellish or freshen your water with lemon, cucumber slices, or even mint leaves. Just don't let liquid cross over from water to tea and you will be okay.

Q. *I see that I should drink filtered water, but does that mean I need to buy bottled water during the fast?*

A. No, you don't need to drink only bottled water, but it is advised to use a filtering pitcher during the fast. These are widely available, and you can usually purchase one for about twenty-five dollars. Filtering your water all the time is a good choice for your health, so you can get a lot of use out of this purchase.

Q. *My Bible says Daniel ate only vegetables and drank only water. But you say that we can also have fruit. Can you help me understand why fruit is okay?*

A. Older translations use the word *pulse* to refer to foods that come from seeds rather than from animals: "Prove thy servants, I beseech thee, ten days; and let them give us pulse to eat, and water to drink" (Daniel 1:12, KJV). Many versions translated *pulse* as "vegetables." However many Bible scholars and commentators, including Matthew Henry, contend that pulse would mean that plant-based foods were given to the Hebrew men.

Q. *Is it okay to exercise and work out during the Daniel Fast?*

A. Yes, it's great to exercise while you fast. However, if you are very active you will want to make sure you are eating enough protein.

If you don't think you are getting enough by eating leafy green vegetables, whole grains, nuts, beans with rice, and soy products, you might want to modify the fast by adding appropriate amounts of fish and chicken.

Q. *What are the best Bible verses to read during the Daniel Fast?*

A. I suggest you read the book of Daniel and concentrate on the character of the Hebrew men who were taken into captivity and yet maintained their deep faith in their God.

Q. *How do I handle a situation when I have to travel or attend a dinner engagement or a special celebration?*

A. First, it's best if you can plan ahead and avoid these situations. You can pack snacks like nuts and rice cakes and carry your own salad dressing. When traveling, you'll find many restaurants have vegetarian or vegan menu items because so many people are on special diets. But you might find yourself in unavoidable situations. In those times, do the best you can and then return to the Daniel Fast guidelines when you return home.

When you go to someone's home for dinner, you might call ahead and tell your host that you are on a temporary special diet and ask for a simple vegetable salad. Or you may need to push the pause button on your fast if that is the most loving way to handle the situation. Be moderate in your eating, eating enough to please your host rather than feed your cravings.

Q. *Is it okay to use red wine vinegar when wine is not allowed on the Daniel Fast?*

A. This is one of the fine-line issues on the Daniel Fast. The small amount of alcohol found in vinegar does not have any inebriating potential. So in this case the red wine is flavoring, and it would be allowed on the Daniel Fast.

Q. *If the only beverage is water, is it okay to drink smoothies? Also, can I add protein powder to my smoothies?*

A. First, smoothies are not considered a beverage. They are a "liquid meal" like soup and therefore would be allowed on the Daniel Fast. Protein powder can be added as long as it conforms to the Daniel Fast guidelines and is free of dairy, sweetener, and chemicals. Look for an unsweetened soy-based protein powder.

Q. *Is it okay to eat apples and rice during the Daniel Fast, since Daniel didn't have access to these foods?*

A. Yes, it's okay to eat these and other foods, as long as they originate from seed. We are not trying to eat only the foods Daniel ate during the fast, but rather we are trying to use the guidelines his fast employed. If apples and rice had been available to Daniel, given the restrictions he established, he would have included them in his diet.

Q. *Is it okay to take medications during the Daniel Fast? Also, what about vitamins and supplements?*

A. A fast should never bring harm to the body, so if your health provider has prescribed medications, then by all means continue taking them during the fast. Likewise, vitamins and supplements are allowed on the fast. If possible, be sure the supplements don't include sweeteners or man-made chemicals.

Q. *I have diabetes and am wondering if the Daniel Fast is safe for me.*

A. You will want to monitor your blood sugar during the Daniel Fast and also make sure you consult with your health provider if eating this way is a great change from your typical diet. However, I have received numerous reports from men and women with diabetes stating that the Daniel Fast has been so beneficial to their health that their blood sugar is balanced and they now are controlling the diabetes through healthy eating. However, if you need to modify the fast to meet your health needs, then that is perfectly acceptable.

Q. *I am having caffeine withdrawals that include headaches, fatigue, and moodiness. How long will this last, and is there anything I can do to relieve the symptoms?*

A. The best thing to do is to taper off caffeine before you begin your fast. However, if that didn't happen, then be sure to drink at least a half gallon of filtered water each day and take 400 mg of vitamin C in the morning and again at dinnertime. Also, long walks seem to lessen the detox symptoms, which usually pass after three to five days. If the symptoms are very severe and you find them significantly interfering with your ability to function, then drink a small amount of coffee and begin tapering off so that within a week you are not drinking any coffee. You can taper off by substituting 50 percent of your coffee with decaffeinated coffee every day until the symptoms are gone. Again, be sure to also drink at least a half gallon of filtered water each day.

Q. *What if I have more questions about the fast?*

A. The best thing to do is to go to http://www.Daniel-Fast.com and click on the "Blog." There you will find thousands of posts from men and women around the world, and most likely you will find the answers to your questions. However, if you still need help just click the "Contact" option and e-mail your question to me.

Acknowledgments

I WANT TO THANK the members of my "life support team" who have invested in and stood alongside me over the years. I am grateful to you and for you! While this list is not exhaustive, I do want to recognize Erin Bishop, Lynn Chittenden, Mick Fleming, Nole Ann Horsey, Sid Kaplan, Michael Main, Tonia Pugel, Lili Salas, Pastors David and Linda Saltzman and Ellensburg Foursquare Church, Pastor Abbie Thela (my little brother-in-love), Fr. Paul Waldie, OMI (a living testimony of Christian love), and my dear children, grandchildren, and family.

This book would likely be sitting on the hard drive of my computer if it wasn't for Ann Spangler, whose wisdom, experience, and giftedness have been priceless. I also want to thank the professional and dedicated team at Tyndale House Publishers—especially my editor, Lisa Jackson.

The foundation of everything good in my life is my amazing Father to whom I am grateful beyond words. Thank You for the conversations and time we spend together, along with the guidance, love, grace, and joy You give so generously. You have shown me comfort, security, and power in the Way, the Truth, and the Life. My sincere hope is to serve You as I serve Your people who use this book to grow in the love, knowledge, and grace of Your Son through the spiritual discipline of prayer and fasting.

Notes

1. *The Daniel Fast* blog, http://www.DanielFast.wordpress.com, and website, http://www.Daniel-Fast.com.
2. Matthew Henry, *Matthew Henry's Complete Commentary on the Whole Bible*, Daniel 1:12, "*Prove us for ten days;* during that time let us have nothing but *pulse to eat,* nothing but herbs and fruits, or parched peas or lentils, and nothing but *water to drink,* and see how we can live upon that, and proceed accordingly."
3. There are two primary theological views of the makeup of humankind. The view that a person is comprised of two parts (body and soul) is called *dichotomy.* The view that a person is comprised of three parts (body, soul, and spirit) is called *trichotomy.* There is also the philosophy of *monism* that says there is no distinction between body and soul. Although I am not a theologian, I believe that Scripture teaches the trichotomy of humankind.
4. Caroline Leaf, *Who Switched Off My Brain?* (Dallas: Switch On Your Brain USA LP, 2009), or see "Thought Life," http://www.drleaf.net/osc/thoughtlife.php?osCsid=3fa ebe66f468b5971458c23060bb4b01 (accessed September 28, 2009).
5. Trust for America's Health, "TFAH Testifies before Congress on America's Obesity Epidemic during Economic Recession," March 26, 2009, http://healthyamericans .org/newsroom/releases/?releaseid=164 (accessed August 12, 2009).
6. World Health Organization, "Diabetes Programme: Facts and Figures," http:// www.who.int/diabetes/facts/world_figures/en/ (accessed September 28, 2009).
7. Peter L. Williams and Roger Warwick, eds., *Gray's Anatomy*, 36th British Edition (Edinburgh/New York: C. Livingstone, 1980), 1350.
8. Mayo Clinic, "Dietary Fiber: An Essential Part of a Healthy Diet," http://www .mayoclinic.com/health/fiber/NU00033.
9. Adapted from http://www.mayoclinic.com/health/high-fiber-foods/NU00582.
10. Mayo Clinic, "Water: How Much Should You Drink Every Day?" http://www .mayoclinic.com/health/water/nu00283 (accessed May 25, 2009).
11. American Heart Association, "Know How Many Calories You Should Eat," http:// www.americanheart.org/presenter.jhtml?identifier=3040366 (accessed September 21, 2009).
12. See http://www.centralbean.com/cooking.html.

Daniel Fast
Recipe Index

About the Author

Susan Gregory, "The Daniel Fast Blogger," launched *The Daniel Fast* blog and website in December 2007. Since then, her site has received millions of hits. Susan is passionate to see individuals experience a successful Daniel Fast as they seek God and endeavor to grow in the love and knowledge of Christ. Author of *Out of the Rat Race*, Susan has written for nationally known ministries and her work has taken her to more than thirty-five countries. A mother and grandmother, she lives on a small farm in Washington State. Visit her online at http://www.Daniel-Fast.com.

Online Discussion *guide*

TAKE *your* TYNDALE READING EXPERIENCE *to the* NEXT LEVEL

A FREE discussion guide for this book is available at bookclubhub.net, perfect for sparking conversations in your book group or for digging deeper into the text on your own.

www.bookclubhub.net

You'll also find free discussion guides for other Tyndale books, e-newsletters, e-mail devotionals, virtual book tours, and more!

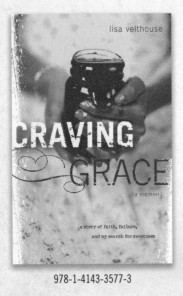

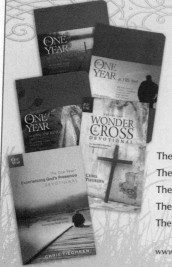

What do you do when God just seems

too far away?

INCLUDES EXERCISES FOR EACH OF THE 9 SPIRITUAL TEMPERAMENTS

WHAT'S YOUR GOD LANGUAGE?

*Connecting with God through
Your Unique Spiritual Temperament*

DR. MYRA PERRINE

FOREWORD BY GARY THOMAS

Many of us find it tough to really feel connected with God. So we try to model what we've seen others do—singing worship songs, engaging in acts of service, meditating quietly in solitude—but since God has designed each of us with a unique personality, we find that one-size-fits-all spirituality just doesn't work.

In *What's Your God Language?* teacher and spiritual director Dr. Myra Perrine will help you discover your own spiritual temperament—the way God has given you to best communicate with Him. As you draw closer to God, you'll learn to love Him in a new way . . . the way you were created to love Him.

CP0226